REFLEX SYMPATHETIC DYSTROPHY

CURRENT MANAGEMENT OF PAIN

P. PRITHVI RAJ. SERIES EDITOR

The series, *Current Management of Pain,* is intended by the series editor and the publishers to provide up-to-date information on advances in the clinical management of acute and chronic pain and related research as quickly as possible. Both the series editor and the publishers felt that, although comprehensive texts are now available, they do not always cover the rapid advances in this field. Another format was needed to publish advances in basic sciences and clinical modalities and to bring them rapidly to the practitioners in the community. A questionnaire was sent to selected clinicians and, based on their responses, topics were chosen by the series editor. Editors of each volume were chosen for their expertise in the field and their ability to encourage other active pain specialists to contribute their knowledge:

Ghia, J.N., ed.: The Multidisciplinary Pain Center: Organization and Personnel Functions for Pain Management, 1988. ISBN 0-89838-359-5. CUMP 1

Lynch, N.T., Vasudevan, S.V.: Persistent Pain: Psychosocial Assessment and Intervention, 1988. ISBN 0-89838-363-3. CUMP 2

Abram, S.E., ed.: Cancer Pain, 1988. ISBN 0-89838-389-7. CUMP 3

Racz, G.B., ed.: Techniques of Neurolysis, 1989. ISBN 0-89838-397-8. CUMP 4

Stanton-Hicks, M., ed.: Pain and the Sympathetic Nervous System, 1989. ISBN 0-7923-0304-0. CUMP 5

Rawal, N., Coombs, D.W., eds.: Spinal Narcotics, 1989. ISBN 0-7923-0374-1. CUMP 6

Stanton-Hicks, M., Jänig, W., Boas, R., eds.: Reflex Sympathetic Dystrophy, 1989. CUMP 7

REFLEX SYMPATHETIC DYSTROPHY

EDITED BY MICHAEL STANTON-HICKS, M.D.,
WILFRID JÄNIG, PH.D., ROBERT A. BOAS, M.D.

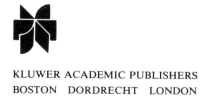

KLUWER ACADEMIC PUBLISHERS
BOSTON   DORDRECHT   LONDON

Printed in the United States of America

Distributors for North America:
Kluwer Academic Publishers
101 Philip Drive
Assinippi Park
Norwell, Massachusetts 02061 USA

Distributors for all other countries:
Kluwer Academic Publishers Group
Distribution Centre
Post Office Box 322
3300 AH Dordrecht, THE NETHERLANDS

Library of Congress Cataloging-in-Publication Data

Reflex sympathetic dystrophy.

  (Current management of pain ; # 7)
  1. Reflex sympathetic dystrophy—Congresses.
I. Stanton-Hicks, Michael d'A.   II. Janig, Wilfrid.
III. Boas, Robert A.   IV. Series.   [DNLM: 1. Reflex
Sympathetic Dystrophy.   W1 CU788LW v.7 / WL 600 R332]
RC422.R43R44   1989   617.5′8   89-24474
ISBN 0-7923-0527-2

CONTENTS

Section II

Section III

Therapeutic Techniques in RSD

viii Contents

Section IV

<u>New Techniques</u>

CONTRIBUTING AUTHORS

Stephen E. Abram, M.D.
Professor
Department of Anesthesia
Medical College of Wisconsin
8700 W. Wisconsin Avenue
Milwaukee, WI 53226

H. Blumberg, M.D.
Abt. für Klinische Neurologie
und Neurophysiologie
Klinikum der Albert-Ludwigs-
Universität, Freiburg

Robert A. Boas, M.D.
Assoc. Professor
Department of Clinical Pharmacology,
University of Auckland
New Zealand (on Sabbatical)
University of Washington
Seattle, WA 98195

Stephen H. Butler, M.D.
Assoc. Professor
Department of Anesthesiology
University of Washington
Seattle, WA 98195

Jeffrey Cannella, M.D.
Assistant Professor of Anesthesiology
University Center for Pain Medicine
at Hermann
University of Texas
Houston, TX 77030

J. E. Charlton, M.D.
Department of Anaesthetics
University of Newcastle
Newcastle, England

U. T. Egle, M.D.
Klinik und Poliklinik fur
Psychosomatische Medizin u.
Psychotherapie
Johannes Gutenberg-Universität
Mainz, F.R.G.

C. J. Glynn, M.D.
Consultant
Oxford Regional Pain Relief Unit
Oxford, England

H. J. Griesser, M.D.
Abt. für Klinische Neurologie
und Neurophysiologie
Klinikum der Albert-Ludwigs-
Universität, Freiburg

J. David Haddox, M.D.
Assistant Professor
Department of Anesthesiology and Psychiatry
Medical College of Wisconsin
Milwaukee, WI 53226

K. Hahn, M.D.
Institut für Klinische Strahlenkunde
Abteilung für Nuklearmedizin
Klinikum der Johannes Gutenberg-Universität Mainz

J. G. Hannington-Kiff, M.D.
Director
Pain Relief Centre
Frimley Park Hospital
England

James E. Heavner, M.D.
Department of Anethesiology
University of Texas
Lubbock, TX

S. O. Hoffman, M.D.
Klinik und Poliklinik für
Psychosomatische Medizin u.
Psychotherapie
Johannes Gutenberg-Universität
Mainz, F.R.G.

M. E. Hornyak
Abt. für Klinische Neurologie
und Neurophysiologie,
Klinikum der Albert-Ludwigs-
Universität, Freiburg

Wilfrid Jänig, Ph.D.
Professor und Leiter
Physiologisches Institut
Christian Albrechts-Universität
Kiel, F.R.G.

Ilmar Jurna, M.D.
Professor und Leiter
Institut für Pharmakologie und
Toxologie, Universität des Saarlandes
Homburg, F.R.G.

Jennifer Kelly, Ph.D.
Assistant Professor Psychology
University Center for Pain Medicine
at Hermann
University of Texas
Houston, TX

Boyce Lewis Jr., M.D.
Department of Anesthesiology
University of Texas
Lubbock, TX

Patricia Lowry, M.D.
Assistant Professor of Radiology
University of Texas
Houston, TX

Karen McConn
Physical Therapy Supervisor
University Center for Pain Medicine
at Hermann
University of Texas
Houston, TX

Terence Murphy, M.D.
Professor
Department of Anesthesiology and
Clinical Pain Service
University of Washington
Seattle, WA

O. Nickel, M.D.
Institut für Klinische Strahlenkunde
Abteilung fur Nuklearmedizin
Klinikum der Johannes Gutenberg-Universität Mainz

Gabor B. Racz, M.D.
Professor and Chairman
Department of Anesthesiology
University of Texas
Lubbock, TX

P. Prithvi Raj, M.D.
Professor of Anesthesiology
Director
University Center for Pain Medicine
at Hermann
University of Texas
Houston, TX

William J. Roberts, Ph.D.
Neurological Sciences Institute
Good Samaritan Hospital and Medical Center
Portland, OR

John Scott, M.D.
Department of Anesthesiology
University of Texas
Lubbock, TX

Michael Stanton-Hicks, M.D.
Professor
Oberarzt für Schmerz und Forschung
Klinik für Anesthesiologie
Johannes Gutenberg-Universität
Mainz, F.R.G.

H. Steinert
Institut für Klinische Strahlenkunde
Abteilung fur Nuklearmedizin
Klinikum der Johannes Gutenberg-Universität Mainz

Ronald R. Tasker, M.D.
Head, Division of Neurosurgery
Toronto General Hospital
Canada

Erik Torebjörk, M.D.
Department of Clinical Neurophysiology
University Hospital
Uppsala, Sweden

Peter R. Wilson, M.D.
Assoc. Professor
Department of Anesthesiology
Mayo Clinic
Rochester, MN

Discussants

B. Edwards, M.D.
Co-Director
Rehabilitation Unit
St. Joseph's Medical Center
South Bend, IN

H. Fruhstorfer, Ph.D.
Professor
Institut für Normale und
Pathologische Physiologie
Phillipps-Universität
3550 Marburg
F.R.G.

U. Gerbershagen, M.D.
Professor and Co-Director
Schmerz Zentrum Mainz, F.R.G.

H. Kruescher, M.D.
Chefarzt, Institut für Anesthesiologie
Stadt. Kliniken Osnabruck
Osnabruck, F.R.G.

H. Nolte, M.D.
Chefarzt, Abt. für Aesthesiologie
Kreiskrankenhaus Minden, F.R.G.

Albert van Steenberge, M.D.
Head, Department of Anesthesia
Klinik St. Anne
Bruxelles, Belgian

M. Zimmerman, M.D.
Professor und Leiter
Physiologisches Institut
Universität Heidelberg
Heidelberg, F.R.G.

SERIES EDITOR FOREWORD

Painful disorders following injury of peripheral nerves, bones and other soft tissues have occurred from the earliest times of human existence. Ambroise Pare was called upon to treat the persistent pain experienced by King Charles IX which was caused by a lancet wound. The pain was persistent, diffuse and associated with contracture of muscles. The king could neither flex nor extend his arm for a month until the pain finally disappeared.

Weir Mitchell, G.R. Moorehouse, and W.W. Keene produced a monumental treatise in 1864 titled "Gunshot Wounds and Other Injuries of Nerves," which contained an account of symptoms and signs of peripheral nerve injuries as observed in Unionist Soldiers. After 1864, however, little mention of this condition was made during peacetime until a spate of articles appeared again after World War One and Two.

With the formation of societies such as International Association for the Study of Pain, renewed interest has been shown in understanding the mechanisms and management of pain syndromes. Pain caused by sympathetic disorders has always caught the fancy of clinicians, and yet confusion exists as to the etiology and proper treatment of reflex sympathetic dystrophy. Many new names have been proposed for these syndromes; recent ones include sympathetically or non sympathetically maintained pain.

Taxonomy of The International Association for the Study of Pain lists causalgia and reflex sympathetic syndromes as two distinct entities. All clinicians seem to feel that pain relieved by a diagnostic sympathetic block should be labeled as causalgia or reflex sympathetic dystrophy. Similarly, numerous therapeutic modalities have been proposed. They all center around sympathetic denervation of some sort, pharmacologically, chemically, or surgically. In spite of a great advance in our understanding of pain mechanism in the last quarter century, we are no closer to improving the outcome of patients with severe reflex sympathetic dystrophy. Etiology and incidence is still unclear. Diagnosis is made late and treatment is not standardized. Clinicians who treat causalgia and reflex sympathetic dystrophy have different treatments based upon their background and experience, rather than on the mechanism of the syndrome itself.

The time is opportune now to gather some unbiased thoughts on RSD and clear the air. Our editors, in particular Michael Stanton-Hicks, need to be congratulated for organizing a timely symposium on the subject and inviting international experts to discuss the pathophysiology and treatment of RSD. What follows in this monograph is a clear, concise presentation and discussion of nomenclature, etiology, incidence, mechanism, treatment, and outcome of RSD.

I have no doubt that the readers will find this new information useful in management of patients with RSD in their daily practice.

PREFACE

The syndrome of Reflex Sympathetic Dystrophy is one long recognized clinically by those providing treatment for chronic pain. Despite this, basic research has been sparse with little support from clinical studies to clarify our understanding of the syndrome or reveal its pathophysiology. While many clinical investigators have added their own diagnostic points and new terminology, confusion rather than consensus now prevails.

Provocative enquiry by recent clinical researchers like P. W. Nathan and J. J. Bonica challenged conventions of the day encouraging much of the momentum in study, which has led to the Workshop and material appearing in this text.

To discuss the syndrome RSD, clinicians and basic scientists drawn from 9 countries gathered at Schloss Rettershof, Kelkheim in West Germany last Fall. In keeping with its present description as a triad of autonomic, motor and sensory disturbances in an extremity following a precipitating event, the participants reviewed RSD against all of the other descriptions that are now assembled under the term sympathetically maintained pain. There was general agreement that the sympathetic nervous system is variably involved with the generation and maintenance of the clinical phenomena of RSD but that the syndrome is probably aneurologic disease.

The charge of the Workshop was an attempt to develop a statement that might more clearly define the syndrome of RSD, provide minimal diagnostic criteria and screening tests as well as confirmatory laboratory methods and to offer guidelines for future epidemiological, basic and clinical research. While the material listed in the table of contents accurately reflects the topics discussed, it may not belie the differing points of view that were expressed throughout the Workshop; the greatest difficulty being what should be included under the term RSD.

We hope also that clinicians will be encouraged to maintain outcome audits of their cases and also that therapists will focus their treatment on multidisciplinary management techniques. At the very least it is hoped that this meeting and its text will consolidate and coordinate efforts of those working in the field of pain and rehabilitation, for patients with posttraumatic painful disorders. More immediate tangible consequences of this Workshop include the formation of a special interest section with the IASP, under whose sponsorship the Workshop was held, and submissions for a redefinition of RSD terminology of the Taxonomy of Pain. A synthesis of these ideas and a suggested definition of RSD can be found at the end of the text.

ACKNOWLEDGEMENTS

The editors are indebted to the generosity of the following firms, without whose support neither the Workshop nor its issue in the form of these Proceedings would have been possible:

Astra Chemicals GmbH F.R.G.
Astra Pain Control, Sodertalje Sweden
Baxter Health Care Corp. Valencia, U.S.A.
Boehringer/Mannheim F.R.G.
B. Braun/Melsungen
Burron Medical Inc., Bethlehem, U.S.A.
Ciba-Geigy BmgH, F.R.G.
Deutsche Wellcome GmbH, F.R.G.
Fresenius A.G. F.R.G.
Godecke A.G. F.R.G.
Gneunthal GmbH, F.R.G.
Medtronic, MI, U.S.A.
Mundipharmia GmbH, F.R.G.
Pharmacia Deltec, Inc. MI, U.S.A.

Section I

GENERAL CONSIDERATIONS

1

REFLEX SYMPATHETIC DYSTROPHY: CLINICAL FEATURES

Stephen H. Butler

INTRODUCTION

In order to discuss the clinical presentation of the disorder Reflex Sympathetic Dystrophy (RSD), a definition of the term is necessary.

The term was first used by Evans in 1946 (5), with reappearance over the next few years in a series of articles in the surgical literature. It was further popularized in the pain literature by Bonica (1), and came to indicate a spectrum of previously distinct syndromes. They have in common, regional pain, vasomotor and integumentary findings of varying severity, up to and including causalgia, a distinct entity following nerve injury. RSD has been defined by the International Association for the Study of Pain (IASP) as: Continuous pain in a portion of an extremity after trauma which may include fracture but does not involve a major nerve, and is associated with sympathetic hyperactivity (14). Although causalgia is left as a separate syndrome, this is arguable since the symptomatology and clinical presentations of the conditions overlap, as do their treatments, and possibly also their pathophysiology.

A review of the clinical syndromes which Bonica (1) grouped under the umbrella term "minor reflex sympathetic dystrophies" gives insight into the clinical presentation of the disorder or syndrome known as RSD:

> Sudeck's atrophy
>
> traumatic arthritis
>
> minor causalgia
>
> posttraumatic osteoporosis

posttraumatic pain syndrome

posttraumatic oedema

posttraumatic angiospasm

shoulder-hand syndrome

Unfortunately, the general definition proposed by the Taxonomy Committee of IASP appears to include some rather surprising clinical cases. A review of the literature from the past two years has revealed 73 citations proposing RSD in areas as diverse as chronic knee pain (3), penile pain (2), and atypical facial pain (8) with treatments ranging from "Scottish baths" to contralateral sympathectomy. Perhaps a better understanding of the entity, its pathophysiology and causes will lead to more accurate diagnosis and appropriate treatment. Much clinical and laboratory research lies ahead as this volume attests.

CLINICAL DESCRIPTIONS

With this vagueness of diagnosis, the clinical descriptions cannot help but be somewhat imprecise, especially when considering mild to severe presentations. The cardinal areas to be considered in the clinical state are: (1) pain, (2) trophic changes, (3) autonomic (vasomotor and sudomotor) instability, (4) sensory abnormalities and (5) bony changes.

1.   Pain

Pain is the most important symptom in RSD from both the patient's and clinician's viewpoint. Classically, the pain has a burning quality, but it may also present as an aching discomfort. It is generally felt in the distal part of a limb, initially in a non-segmental distribution. If the symptoms persist, the pain becomes more diffuse, gradually spreading proximally to involve the limb girdle. It may then involve the contralateral limb and has even been described as occurring in the other ipsilateral limb. This spreading discomfort is usually of an aching quality, especially when it involves limb girdles and other limbs (12).

The pain usually appears soon after injury, although some authors describe a delay (13,1). Its intensity is variable, from a mild dull sensation to severe burning which interferes with sleep and all activity. Some patients also describe paroxysmal pain, although the norm is for pain to be steady, no matter the level.

2.   Trophic changes

Trophic changes occur most obviously in the integu mentary system, but are prominent in the musculoskeletal system as well. Local brawny edema is often the first notable change in skin, with gradual thickening and coarsening of the skin over days to a few weeks. Then the skin gradually thins, loses its normal wrinkles and becomes smooth and tight. Hair coarsens and the nails become thickened, ridged, and brittle.

As this process occurs, muscle shortening, atrophy and weakness takes place, as does stiffening to ankylosis of the local and then the regional joints. Those most affected are the metacarpal/metatarsal-phalangeal joints with more distal and then later more proximal joints being involved (9). Patchy osteoporosis is a parallel process (10).

Regional changes with muscle stiffness, soreness and classical myofascial findings spread from the distal limb to the limb girdle, to the contralateral limb, and then become more diffuse. These changes are almost universally seen and present within the first two weeks (16). If unchecked, these may lead to more generalized ankylosis with joint changes as in the shoulder-hand syndrome (17).

3. Autonomic instability

Vasomotor instability is an unusual phenomenon which led early recorders of the disease to implicate the sympathetic nervous system in the pathophysiology of the RSD syndrome.

Classically, the dystrophic limb is cool, pale or cyanotic and sweaty, indicating sympathetic hyperactivity. This state may not occur until days or weeks after the initiating event or onset of problems. The limb may also be warm, red, or suffused and dry. Bonica (1) and Livingston (12) stated that this is usually an early feature of RSD, although later writers disagree (15), perhaps because patients were seen at a later stage. Sudomotor changes tend to parallel vasomotor responses. In the early phases, skin dryness may dominate, but as cutaneous vasoconstriction occurs so too does the development of increased sweating and trophic change.

4. Sensory abnormalities

Dysesthesia and allodynia (to cold and to mechanical stimuli) are variable accompaniments of RSD; especially prominent in severe cases. They are more frequent in causalgia, i.e., where nerve damage has occurred, but nerve damage is not necessarily a preceding event. These sensory abnormalities are not always dermatomal in their distribution, spreading regionally in time to present over most of the affected limb.

5. Bony changes

Gradual roentgenographic and scintigraphic changes evolve through the course of RSD in the majority of cases. They are often overlooked but can be used as a guide to evolution and/or response to treatment. Kozin's articles (9,10,11) are more recent updates on the information first outlined by Sudeck (18) and Fontaine and Herrmann (6).

As mentioned briefly in the description of trophic changes, initially a patchy osteoporosis appears in juxta-articular bone of the affected limb. This begins in the metacarpal-phalangeal or metatarsal-phalangeal joints, but spreads to involve more proximal and distal joints. A more generalized osteoporosis appears as does erosion of subchondral bone of these joints. Scintigraphy using technetium radionuclides in static and flow studies show asymmetry with increased periarticular uptake and flow on the affected side. Kozin et al., felt that scintigraphy was more sensitive than plain films in making the diagnosis of RSD (11). (See (7) for a detailed report of all radiological findings.) More recent developments in three phase bone scanning have added further specificity to RSD diagnosis and are detailed further in Chapter 18.

The onset and course of RSD varies, depending on the precipitating event and its progression, the response of the individual to the precipitating event, and the treatments both for the RSD and/or any underlying disease process. As with so many other chronic pain syndromes and problems, we do not understand what triggers the onset of RSD in any one individual.

THE THREE STAGES OF RSD

The course of RSD was initially defined in three stages by De Takats (4) with later modifications by Bonica (1). Obviously, the process of evolution is a continuum rather than a series of finite steps, so that staging assists only in making some approximation of severity and therefore helps determine treatment intensity.

Stage I (mild)

Beginning within days to a few weeks of the precipi tating event, this stage is characterized by pain, often burning, in the area of the injury. There is frequently hyperesthesia as well. Movement worsens pain and the immobility of the limb is obvious from its protective position. There is usually an accompanying edema, tenderness of the distal joints of the limb and often local muscle spasm as well. The limb may be either warm, red and dry, or cool and pale. Roentgenological examination may show some spotty osteoporosis in peri-articular areas of the bones of the hands or feet. This stage may resolve spontaneously, or respond rapidly to any appropriate treatment modality. The duration of this clinical picture varies from days to a few months.

Stage II (moderate)

As the RSD process progresses, pain can be increased, decreased or unchanged. There may be the beginning of local hyperesthesia, paresthesia and allodynia. Edema spreads and local joints become stiff. Muscle wasting in the region of injury begins, and myofascial findings progress to involve the ipsilateral and contralateral limb girdles. The skin is cold, pale to cyanotic, and moist. The hair of the affected limb becomes thickened and coarse, as do the nails. Osteoporosis progresses to a diffuse form (two to six weeks from onset) and increased technetium uptake by scintigraphy is seen. Appropriate treatments can still be effective, although the response is less brisk and abnormalities may persist for months.

Stage III (severe)

This final stage is marked by severe trophic changes and resistance to treatment. The pain is variable, but often increased. Spreading allodynia and dysesthesiae are frequently part of the pain complaints. Aside from the burning discomfort, there is often a regional aching or throbbing component. Exposure to colds or drafts may aggravate the pain. Extreme immobility of the limb is present, partly because of progressive ankylosis of the joints, and partly due to atrophy and contracture of muscles. Edema has resolved and the subcutaneous tissue has become atrophied. The skin is smooth, thin and shiny, cold and often damp. The nails and hair become coarse, thickened and brittle. These patients are often anxious, tentative and depressed with all the vegetative symptoms of that state. Radiological examinations show diffuse osteoporosis and increased flow by scan. Treatment is less likely to be helpful because of the seemingly permanent nature of many of these changes.

SUMMARY

This chapter has reviewed the clinical presentation of RSD on the basis of previous descriptions of the syndrome colored by some personal bias. Since the guidelines for diagnosis are vague and as the clinical course of the RSD process is highly variable with spontaneous remission possible, the basis for clinical assessment and therapy of the syndrome is not clear. This makes for great difficulty in evaluating treatment outcomes, and is probably why so varied a range of "appropriate" treatments exists.

It is hoped that a greater understanding of RSD as might arise from these further papers and their discussions, will allow more precise diagnosis and treatment for the benefit of those suffering from this condition.

REFERENCES

1.   Bonica, J.J. The management of pain. Lea and Febiger, 1953.

2.   Chalkey, J.E., et al. Probable reflex sympathetic dystrophy of the penis. Pain, 25 (2): 223-225, 1986.

3.   Coughlin, R.J., et al. Algodystrophy: A common unrecognized cause of chronic knee pain. Br J Rheumatol, 26 (4): 270-274, 1987.

4.   De Takats, G. Reflex dystrophy of the extremities. Arch Surg, 34: 939, 1937.

5.   Evans, J.A. Reflex sympathetic dystrophy. Surg Clin N A, 26: 780, 1946.

6.   Fontaine, R., Herrmann, L. Posttraumatic osteoporosis. Ann Surg, 17: 26, 1933.

7.   Genant, H.K., et al. The reflex sympathetic dystrophy syndrome: A comprehensive analysis using fine-detail radiography, photon adsorptometry, and bone and joint scintigraphy. Radiology, 117: 21, 1975.

8.   Jaeger, B., Singer, E., Kroening, R. Reflex sympathetic dystrophy of the face. Report of two cases and a review of the literature. Arch Neurol., 43 (7): 693-695 1986

9.   Kozin, F., et al. The reflex sympathetic dystrophy syndrome II. Roentgenographic and scintigraphic evidence of bilaterality and of periarticular accentuation. Am J Med, 60: 332-338, 1976.

10.   Kozin, F., et al. The reflex sympathetic dystrophy syndrome I. Clinical and histological studies: evidence for bilaterality, response to cortico steroids and articular involvement. Am J Med, 60:321-331 1976

11.   Kozin, F., et al. The reflex sympathetic dystrophy syndrome (RSDS) III. Scintigraphic studies, further evidence for the therapeutic efficacy of systemic corticosteroids, and proposed diagnostic criteria. Am J Med, 70: 23-30, 1981.

12.   Livingston, W.K. Pain mechanisms. Macmillan, 1943.

13.   Mitchell, S.W., et al. Gunshot wounds and other injuries of nerves.
        J. B. Lippincott & Co., 1864.

14.   Pain, Supp 3, S29, 1986.

15.   Schumacker, H.B., Abramson, D.I. Posttraumatic vasomotor
        disorders. Surg Gynec & Obst, 88: 417, 1949.

16.   Sola, A. Personal communication.

17.   Steinbrocker, O. The shoulder-hand syndrome. Am J Med, 3: 403,
        1947.

18.   Sudeck, P. Ueber die acute enzundliche knochenatropie. Arch Klin
        Chir, 62: 147, 1900.

2

REFLEX SYMPATHETIC DYSTROPHY:
INCIDENCE AND EPIDEMIOLOGY

Stephen E. Abram

There is relatively little information available regarding the overall incidence of causalgia and reflex sympathetic dystrophy (RSD) in the general population. Carron and Weller (1) reported that they documented 123 patients, who met rigid criteria for RSD among 1156 pain clinic patients (10.7%) treated over a 22-month period. Unfortunately, it is impossible to determine the population base from which those patients came. Sixty-three percent of those patients had upper extremity involvement. We diagnosed RSD in 41 of 653 patients (6.3%) admitted to the Medical College of Wisconsin Pain Clinic (unpublished data). Seventy-three percent of those cases occurred in the upper extremity. Other series also show a tendency for the syndrome to occur in the upper extremity, at least in adult patients (2,3). Bonica (4) reported that two thirds of cases of causalgia (associated with major nerve trunk injury) involved the upper extremity.

Although discussions of predisposition to RSD often mention such terms as the "typical RSD personality" or underlying psychopathology, there is little evidence to support such notions. Haddox (5), using the McGill and Dartmouth questionnaires and the State Trait Anxiety Inventory, was unable to demonstrate any differences between a group of tightly selected RSD patients and a group of patients with radiculopathy. He discusses the psychological aspects of RSD in detail in chapter 15 in this text. Another study failed to reveal any personality differences between a group of RSD patients and a group of patients with nerve injuries without evidence of RSD (6).

The ratio of males to females with RSD varies considerably from one series to the next. In our study at the Medical College of Wisconsin, 61% of RSD patients were women. In Carron's series (1), male patients outnumbered female patients by 2:1, perhaps reflecting the predominance of industrial injuries in that population. In a series published by Kleinert, male patients represented 55% of cases (7), while in two other series about two thirds of the patients were women (8,9). It has been reported that RSD is most prevalent among women over the age of 50 (10). Kleinert noted that a relatively small percentage of the patients in his series were black (7). Rothberg et al. (11) reported a much higher incidence of causalgia among nerve injured patients above the age of 35 than was seen in patients under age 35 with similar injuries. Both Kleinert (7) and Pak (8) report a predominance of RSD patients between the ages of 40 and 60, with few cases occurring in patients under 30 or over 70.

The term causalgia, often used synonymously with reflex sympathetic dystrophy, is now generally used to specify a syndrome of burning pain, hyperalgesia, vasomotor and sudomotor alterations, and dystrophy occurring after major nerve trunk injury. The great majority of causalgia cases occur after gunshot wounds, most of which are proximal to the knee or elbow. The great majority of cases are related to injuries, usually partial transsections, of the medial cord of the brachial plexus, median nerve or sciatic nerve (4). The great majority of reported cases involved wartime series.

The term reflex sympathetic dystrophy encompasses a symptom complex including that of causalgia, as discussed in Chapter 1, but with a wide range of precipitating injuries and conditions. Bonica (4) has published an extensive list of conditions that have been known to trigger the pathological process. The list includes trauma such as sprains, fractures, lacerations, crush injuries, amputations and burns; surgery; occupational factors, such as repetitive microtrauma and pneumatic tool operation; and a variety of disease states, such as myocardial infarction, neurologic diseases, infection, and vascular disease.

Blunt trauma is the leading cause of RSD in several series (7,8), while fractures tend to be the leading cause in others (1). Wrist fractures are commonly associated with the development of RSD, perhaps because of the frequent association of this injury to injury of the median nerve, which carries most of the sympathetic fibers to the hand. In Kleinert's series (7), well over half of the post-surgical cases of RSD occurred following carpal tunnel surgery or release of a Dupuytren's contracture.

In the RSD literature published prior to 1960, myocardial infarction was a relatively common precipitating factor. Luisada (12) reported the incidence of shoulder hand syndrome following myocardial infarction to be as high as 10 to 15%. In 1943, Johnson (13) reported 39 patients with dystrophy of the hand among 178 consecutive myocardial infarction cases, 34 of whom also reported shoulder pain. A review of four series published since 1970 shows only 2% of RSD cases occurred after myocardial infarction (1,7,8,14). In a recent review of RSD, Schwartzman and McLellan (15) state that the occurrence of RSD following myocardial infarction had dropped to less than 1%. Perhaps the lower incidence is associated with more aggressive pain management, and earlier mobilization and rehabilitation after myocardial infarction.

There is at least some data available regarding the incidence of causalgia following nerve injury. Schwartzman and McLellan (15) cite an incidence ranging from 1 to 15% among nerve injured patients. Bonica, reviewing a number of published series, cites 296 causalgia cases among 12,335 patients with peripheral nerve injuries, an incidence of 2.4% (4). Echlin et al. (16) reported that nearly 20% of patients with nerve injuries reported at least transient symptoms of causalgia. However, only 2% of those patients had symptoms persisting longer than a few days. Richards (17) reviewed several studies of causalgia conducted during World War II. He found that 3.9% of nearly 10,000 nerve injured patients developed the syndrome. Bonica's review (4) showed that 82% of cases involved the brachial plexus, median, sciatic or tibial nerves. Richards (17) reported very similar data, with 83% of 461 cases involving the median or tibial nerves or their components, nerves that carry most of the sympathetic fibers to the hand or foot.

Until very recently, RSD was considered to be a rare syndrome among children. In 1978, Bernstein (18) reported on 23 children who developed RSD. This report appeared in the pediatric literature, and was not widely read by physicians who often deal with the syndrome. Besides the pediatric age range, there were other differences between the patients in that series and the typical adult RSD patients. There were few reports of antecedent trauma among Bernstein's patients, they were predominantly female, and antecedent stress and anxiety was present in many of the patients. Blau (19) reported on a series of 10 pediatric RSD patients, ranging in age from 8 to 17. There was only one male in the group, and as in Bernstein's report, there were few cases that involved antecedent trauma. Most patients exhibited diminished skin temperature in the affected limb early in the course of the disease. This finding differs from many series of adult patients that report warmth and flushing of the affected limb in early RSD. In both series, most patients responded well to physical therapy. In Blau's series the upper and lower limbs were affected with equal frequency.

Goldsmith et al. (20) reported on a series of 15 pediatric RSD patients, ranging in age from 9 to 18. Again, antecedent trauma was uncommon. There was a predominance of males in the group, and 80% involved the lower extremity. None of the patients in that series were black despite a sizeable black population locally. The youngest patients reported with RSD have been 3 years old (21,22). An extensive review of the literature on childhood RSD has revealed approximately 100 cases (18-27).

REFERENCES

1. Carron, H., Weller R.W. Treatment of post-traumatic sympathetic dystrophy. In Advances in neurology, Vol. 4, New York, Raven Press, pp. 485-490, 1974.

2. Patman, D., Thompson, J, Person, A. Management of post-traumatic pain syndrome: Report of 113 cases. Ann Surg, 177: 780-787, 1973.

3. Rosen, P.S., Graham, W. The shoulder hand syndrome: Historical review with observations on seventy-three patients. Can Med Ass J, 77: 86-91, 1958.

4. Bonica, J.J. The management of pain. Philadelphia, Lea and Febiger, p. 948, 1953.

5. Haddox, J.D., Abram, S.E., Hopwood, M.H. Comparison of psychometric testing in RSD and radiculopathy. Regional Anesthesia, 13(1S): 27, 1983.

6. Wilson, R.L. Management of pain following peripheral nerve injuries. Orthop Clin North Am, 12: 343-359, 1981.

7. Kleinert, H.E., Cole, N.M., Wayne, L. et al. Post-traumatic sympathetic dystrophy. Orthop Clin North Am, 4: 917-927, 1973.

8. Pak, T.J., Martin, G.M., Magness, J.L. et al. Reflex sympathetic dystrophy. Minn Med, 53: 507-512, 1970.

9. Drucker W.B., Hubay, C.A., Holden, W.D. et al. Pathogenesis of post-traumatic sympathetic dystrophy. Am J Surg, 97: 454-465, 1959.

10. Steinbroker, O., Argyros, T.G. The shoulder hand syndrome: Present status as a diagnostic and therapeutic entity. Med Clin North Am, 42: 1533-1553, 1958.

11. Rothberg J.M., Tahmoush A.J., Oldakowski, R. The epidemiology of causalgia among soldiers wounded in Viet Nam. Milit Med, 148: 347-350, 1983.

12. Luisada A.A.: Physical therapy in cardiovascular disease. Clinical Cardiology Therapy, 4: 19-94, 1959.

13. Johnson, A.C. Disabling changes in the hand resembling sclerodactylia following myocardial infarction. Ann Int Med, 19: 433-439, 1943.

14. Kozin, F., Ryan, L.M., Carrera, G.F. et al. The reflex sympathetic dystrophy syndrome (RSDS): III. Scintigraphic studies, further evidence for

the therapeutic efficacy of systemic corticosteroids, and proposed diagnostic criteria. Am J Med, 70: 23-30, 1981.

15. Schwartzman, R.J., McLellan, T.L. Reflex sympathetic dystrophy. A review. Arch Neurol, 44: 555-561, 1987.

16. Echlin, F., Owens, F.M., Wells, W.L. Observations of "major" and "minor" causalgia. J Nerv. Ment. Dis., 107: 174-180, 1948.

17. Richards, R.L. Causalgia. A centennial review. Arch Neurol, 16: 339-350, 1967.

18. Bernstein, B.H., Singsen, B.H., Kent, J.T. et al. Reflex neuromuscular dystrophy in childhood. J Pediatr, 93: 211-215, 1978.

19. Blau, E.B. Reflex sympathetic dystrophy syndrome in children. Wis Med J, 83: 34-35, 1984.

20. Goldsmith, D., Feldman, N., Heyman, S. et al. Nuclear imaging in childhood reflex neurovascular dystrophy (CRND). Arthritis Rheum, 29: S92, 1986.

21. Richlin, D.M., Carron, H., Rowlingson, J.C. et al. Reflex sympathetic dystrophy: successful treatment by transcutaneous nerve stimulation. J Pediatr, 93: 84-5, 1978.

22. Kozin, F., Haughton, V., Ryan, L. The reflex sympathetic dystrophy syndrome in a child. J Pediatr, 90: 417-419, 1977.

23. Hayden, P.W., Bolton, R.W. Bone scintigraphy in childhood reflex sympathetic dystrophy. J Nucl Med, 27: 932, 1986.

24. Ilowite, N.T., Lightman, H.I., Pochaczevsky, R. Thermography in Reflex sympathetic dystrophy. Arthritis Rheum, 30: S80, 1987.

25. Laxer, R.M., Allen, R.C., Malleson, P.N. et al. Reflex neurovascular dystrophy in children. Arthritis Rheum, 27: S18, 1984.

26. Ruggeri, S.B., Athreya, B.H., Doughty, R. et al. Reflex sympathetic dystrophy in children. Clin Orthop, 163: 225-230. 1982.

27. Nickeson, R., Brewer, E., Person, D.A. Early histologic and radionuclide scan changes in children with reflex sympathetic dystrophy syndrome (RSDS). Arthritis Rheum, 28: S72, 1985.

3

CHRONIC PAIN MECHANISMS

Terence M. Murphy

Pain has afflicted patients and frustrated therapists since time began. Renewed interest and effort in the management of pain in recent decades (1), and an improved understanding of its complex mechanisms and its multidimensional nature (2) have led to an explosion of scientific and therapeutic interest in pain and its treatment. Renewal of interest in RSD being a case in point. However, before discussing management, it is important to briefly review our current understanding of the nature of pain.

Pain is difficult to define. Virtually all patients (and most physicians) believe it to be due to "nociception." This is the transmission of signals of tissue damaging energy (or potentially damaging energy) along A delta and C fibers of the sensory nervous system to discrete pathways within the neuraxis, with specific projections to the sensory cortex. This mechanism of pain has been long promulgated and lead to a variety of treatments in the pharmacological and neurodestructive arena. Subsequently, experience has taught us that these techniques are more effective for acute than for chronic pain.

While this "straight through" system of "nociception" almost certainly operates in the majority of acute pain situations, it is much less applicable as pain becomes more chronic. The "direct" pathway from peripheral receptor to sensory cortex becomes modified by interaction of this incoming signal, both with other non-nociceptive incoming signals and with descending inhibitory or faciliatory effects from other neurons. In this way, the initial nociceptive signal is subject to wide modification from its origin at the peripheral receptor (1). The final effect can thus be enigmatic, such as an individual with obvious trauma (e.g., injured soldiers in battle, or sports players) who may suffer significant nociception but show no evidence of "pain." Conversely, there are those individuals who present to the medical profession with a plethora of pain symptoms, yet despite investigation, reveal no evidence of nociceptive tissue damage. Such patients pose a great diagnostic and therapeutic challenge to physicians, and are frequently encountered in pain clinic populations.

Patients presenting to pain clinics have chronic pain complaints that can span the whole spectrum from an extensive malignant tumor to a predominant and maybe even exclusively behavioral problem. In these latter cases the behavioral complaint of pain can be so reinforced by environmental circumstances that secondary pain and abnormal behaviors persist long after the original nociceptive damage has resolved.

Pain clinics evolved out of the need to deal with this wide spectrum of patient presentations.

CLASSIFICATION OF CHRONIC PAIN

Although still incompletely understood, a general classification can be made based on the present understanding, whereby chronic pain has been divided into four broad categories, i.e., nociception, central pain states, psychological pain, and behavioral pain, which are defined briefly as follows (2).

1. **Nociception.** This is pain originating usually from tissue damage or threatened damage transmitted via the A delta and C fibers in the afferent sensory nervous system. This is the mechanism for pain which most physicians were taught, and includes the pain of injury, cancer, chronic degenerative arthritic diseases, etc. It tends to respond to conventional analgesia therapies, and is perhaps the best understood of all the mechanisms of pain.

Syndromes of RSD pain fall only partly in this category, probably being initiated by local injury or disease in most cases.

2. **Central pain states.** Here, the pain arises in denervated areas (e.g., phantom limb pain, post stroke pain, probably tic douloureux). Although imperfectly understood, pain may arise as a result of abnormal signal generation in the central nervous system, whereby the message of "nociception" is generated such that the brain receives messages as though nociception were occurring in the periphery when it is not. This type of pain responds poorly if at all to conventional analgesics. Later stages of RSD appear to have a central component to their pain. (See Chapter 6.)

3. **Psychological pain.** Here, the patient uses language and behavior as though nociception were occurring in response to what are believed to be psychological forms of suffering, such as anxiety, depression, neurosis, hysteria, etc. This is probably a very important aspect in many of the chronic entrenched pain patients, and alas, often frequently overlooked in the initial evaluation and prescription of treatment. This "psychogenic" pain cannot be diagnosed by exclusion, but from positive findings acquired by formal psychological and neuropsychiatric evaluation which should be carried out in parallel with physical evaluation. Treatment is usually lengthy with psychological and psychiatric counseling, and psychoactive drugs if needed.

Although controversial in the context of RSD disorders, there may be some contribution in terms of the personality type, to development of passivity in response to injury, as presented by Egle and Hoffmann in Chapter 5 of this text.

4. **Behavioral pain.** Pain is a private sensation. It is communicated as a behavior, i.e., limping, grimacing, complaining, going to doctors, etc. Such responses are the outward means by which we asses the nature of the underlying pain complaint and help provide both the organic diagnosis and the effect of pain on the individual. However, if this behavior is overly reinforced by environmental influences in the social, domestic or employment arena, then the "learned behavior" can outlast the healing process, and persist purely as a behavioral phenomenon. This is believed to be a potent generator in a

significant percent of those patients suffering from chronic pain who fail to respond to conventional anti-nociceptive treatment measures. Treatment of this type of pain must be directed along behavioral modification lines, educating the patient and his immediate social circle as to the nature of the disability (or lack of same), and encouragement and reinforcement of productive rather than pain behavior.

This principal is no less important in the treatment of RSD than other chronic pain states, and is a common default in therapy when directing care of the more severe and resistant cases.

DIAGNOSIS OF CHRONIC PAIN

Most chronic pain patients, including those with RSD, display various aspects of some or all of the above generators. Thus it is important at an early stage, to evaluate and assess the relative contributions of the above factors to an individual's pain complaint, and offer treatment accordingly.

This evaluation is usually done by both a medical examination and a coincident psychological and behavioral analysis of the patient, so the patient and his environment are comprehensively assessed (4). With all the above information in hand, treatment can be applied appropriately to each aspect of the patient's disorder, and conducted in the best sequence to achieve optimal results.

TREATMENT OF CHRONIC PAIN

It is very important to accept the patient's pain complaint as real, and not challenge the existence of pain. Trying to tell a patient that his pain is "imaginary" or "all in his head" rarely helps, but only encourages the patient to seek more and more consultations in an attempt to validate the suffering he feels.

The treatment spectrum for chronic pain can run the whole gamut from selective finite neurodestructive procedure (e.g., celiac plexus blocking in cancer of the pancreas), through to involved psychological behavioral support which may go on over months or years. It should be born in mind, that with our incomplete understanding of pain, it is often impossible to provide total or quick cure for the patient's problem, and that the treatment may well involve a long-term maintenance commitment by both the patient and the physician; in which case family members will usually be included in the therapeutic effort (4).

MEDICATION TREATMENT FOR RSD

Other than the use of non-narcotic analgesics (e.g., aspirin, acetaminophen, NSAIDs) and steroids, there would appear little support for using opiate analgesics other than to facilitate physiotherapy, and then only when other measures have failed or are contra-indicated. However, oral methadone can be useful in stabilizing a patient who has a dependency problem with narcotics when first seen. The patient can be weaned safely and effectively, by initially substituting a therapeutically equivalent dose of methadone (Table 1) in a masking vehicle, and gradually reducing the dose within the masking vehicle as more appropriate treatment strategies are introduced. A similar technique can be used for those patients with a dependency on the sedative hypnotics, whereby phenobarbital is used as a long-acting substitute for the shorter acting sedative hypnotics such as benzodiazepines, etc. (see Table 2) (2).

TABLE 1. Equipotent Analgesic Doses (MGMS)
Of Narcotic Medications

	I.M.	P.O.
Methadone (Dolophine)	7.5	10
Morphine Sulphate	10	60
Diacetylmorphine (Heroin)	3	10
Hydromorphone (Dilaudid)	1.5	7.5
Oxymorphone (Numorphan)	1.5	6
Oxycodone (Percodan)	15	30
Meperidine (Demerol-Petridine)	100	300
Codeine	130	200
*Pentazocine (Talwin)	60	180

*Narcotic antagonist

TABLE 2. Equipotent Doses (MGMS)
Of Sedative-Hypnotic Medications

	P.O.
Phenobarbital	30
Secobarbital (Seconal)	100
Pentobarbital (Nembutal)	100
Diazepam (Valium)	10
Chlordiazapoxide (Librium)	25
Meprobamate (Equanil Miltown)	400
Glutethimide (Doriden)	500
Alcohol (Whiskey)	3 (oz.)

As well as conventional analgesics, patients with depressive or anxiety aspects to their pain complaints may well may need psychoactive medications such as non-dependency producing sedatives (e.g., hydroxyzine or diphenhydramine) and/or the antidepressants.

The tricyclic antidepressants have been much used in recent years in chronic pain therapy to provide nocturnal sedation and sleep in a group of patients who traditionally have had great difficulty in adhering to a normal diurnal rhythm. These drugs may also have an analgesic effect in chronic as opposed to acute pain, but this thesis still needs to be validated. These drugs are very useful therapeutic agents in chronic pain patients (5).

STIMULATION PRODUCED ANALGESIA

This method is most effective using transcutaneous electrical nerve stimulators, which are small portable battery units that enable patients to administer this form of analgesia "around the clock." They help in approximately 30% of chronic pain problems. There may be a place for this therapy during the rehabilitation process in some patients with RSD.

SYMPATHETIC BLOCKS

In RSD the mechanisms for pain production are poorly understood but are characterized by changing patterns of sympathetic activity as described by Jänig

(Chapter 6) and Blumberg et al. (Chapter 10). Injection of the sympathetic ganglia can be very effective in recent onset RSD. In those patients who have a diffuse dysesthetic pain associated with impaired vascular perfusion of an extremity, then diagnostic sympathetic block (either stellate ganglion blocks for the arm or lumbar sympathetic block for the leg) is warranted. This is described in detail in Chapter 11. If good results are obtained, then such treatment should be coupled with active physical therapy during the period the block is effective.

As with all painful conditions, the longer this condition remains untreated, the more social and behavioral influences come to play, the more refractory it is to treatment.

PSYCHOLOGICAL THERAPIES

Many chronic non-malignant patients as mentioned earlier have significant psychological and/or behavioral problems, and if an initial diagnosis suggests an important influence of these factors, then they must be attended to in any subsequent treatment plan (4). Otherwise the treatments outlined above will be less effective. The spectrum of therapies here can vary from the prescribing of some appropriate psychoactive agent, e.g., tranquilizers, antidepressants, etc., through to intensive behavioral modification programs of several weeks duration. In these treatments patients "unlearn" their pain by a combination of educational efforts and physical therapy programs, to become reactivated and demonstrate to both the patients and their spouses the lack of significant "functional impediment." These programs are often effective, even though they may only have a modest reduction in the pain complaint itself. They are also able to achieve considerable reduction in utilization of total health care services (7).

CONCLUSION

The varieties of therapies available for chronic pain and for reflex sympathetic dystrophy as a pertinent example, reflect the current multidimensional model for chronic pain mechanisms. The lack of success of these therapies in a significant number of patients, probably reflects our current imperfect understanding of the mechanisms involved in producing RSD and other pain disorders. As knowledge improves in this area, with basic research and through meetings and reports such as this, we can hopefully look forward to better treatments and improved results for the future.

REFERENCES

1. Melzack, R., Wall, P.D. Pain mechanisms. A new theory. Science, 150: 971-979, 1965.

2. Murphy, T.M. Treatment of chronic pain. In Miller, Anesthesia, 2nd ed., Churchill-Livingstone, 22: 2077-2109, 1986.

3. Boas, R.A. The sympathetic nervous system and pain relief. In Swerdlow (ed.), Relief intractable pain. New York, Elsevier, pp. 215-237, 1983.

4. Fordyce, W.F. Behavioral methods for chronic pain and illness. St. Louis, C.V. Mosby, 1976.

5. Butler, S.H. Present status of tricyclic antidepressants in chronic pain therapy. In Benedetti, C., Chapman, C.R., Morrica, G. (eds.), Recent advances in pain research and therapy, Vol. 7. New York, Raven Press, pp. 177-192, 1986.

4

SYMPATHETICALLY MAINTAINED PAIN
PRINCIPLES OF DIAGNOSIS AND THERAPY

Peter R. Wilson

INTRODUCTION

The role of the sympathetic nervous system (SNS) has not been defined in acute, chronic or neuropathic pain states. However, there seems to be a significant component in reflex sympathetic dystrophy (RSD) and causalgia. There might be a component in such other neuropathic pain states as postherpetic neuralgia, radiculopathies, certain peripheral neuropathies, and central pain syndromes. The role of the SNS is even less clear in conditions such as phantom pain and pain-dysfunction syndromes (PDS). This is a group of poorly-defined pain syndromes which have many of the clinical characteristics of RSD. They include categories such as Repetitive Strain Injury (RSI), Cumulative Trauma Disorder (CTD), Regional Pain Syndrome or Overuse Syndrome (particularly in musicians). They are characterized by progressive pain (often of a burning nature) throughout the extremity, impairment of function, edema, sensory changes and autonomic dysfunction. As described by Roberts (8) and presented later in Chapter 7, these may represent a group better designated as having sympathetically maintained pain, or they may reflect some abnormality in spinal cord signal processing.

DIAGNOSIS OF SYMPATHETIC PAIN SYNDROMES

This syndrome has three stages: (1) Acute hyperemia, (2) Dystrophic ischemia, and (3) Chronic atrophia, and three degrees of severity as presented in the opening chapter: (1) Mild, (2) Moderate, and (3) Severe.

There is therefore no single test or group of tests which are absolutely specific or reliable. The diagnosis is often made by clinical experience and gestalt, in the absence of validated diagnostic criteria. The IASP Taxonomy (2) has proven inadequate and will require redefinition, though the following criteria are suggested as the basis for future standardisation.

Presentation:

1) Burning pain

2) Allodynia

3) Temperature/color changes

4) Edema

5) Skin, hair, nail growth changes

Clinical Tests:

6) Thermometry/thermography

7) Bone x-ray

8) 3-phase bone scan

9) Quantitative sweat test (QSART, cobalt blue)

10) Quantitative sensory testing (cold and mechanical)

11) Response to sympathetic blockade

It is suggested that at least 6 of these criteria are required for a positive diagnosis of RSD. Those with a score of 3-5 may represent "Possible RSD" or fall into the category of "Sympathetically Maintained Pain" where the dystrophic and motor responses are not yet evident. RSD is not present with less than 3 of these criteria. Muscle strength, endurance, and joint mobility in the affected limb should be measured before treatment as a baseline to judge response to treatment. Limb volume measures can be used for the same purpose. In addition, a full medical and work history, social, legal, psychologic and domestic factors must be defined as stressed in the preceding chapter. Ancillary measurements might include EMG and peripheral blood flow studies. Quantitative pain intensity scoring should be objectively evaluated in every case.

TREATMENT

Evaluation of therapy is difficult because of the lack of diagnostic criteria and objective measures of stage and severity of the syndromes. However, rehabilitation of the patient will involve multiple therapeutic interventions.

Physical Therapy

The changes of disuse must be reversed by aggressive active and passive physical therapy.

Disuse causes loss of muscle tone, strength and endurance, atrophy and contractures of muscles, loss of joint mobility, contractures of ligaments, loss of bone calcium, changes in peripheral sensation, and reduction in blood flow.

Physical therapy is essential in reversing these changes, and all ancillary therapy is directed towards facilitating this physical therapy.

Sympathetic Blockage

Sympathetic blockade improves blood flow, and reduces any sympathetic component of the pain. It does not necessarily alter peripheral sensation. *It should only be used in conjunction with appropriate physical therapy.*

Somatic Blockade

In some cases, sympathetic block alone will not provide adequate pain relief to allow adequate physical therapy. Appropriate repeated temporary somatic block may allow improved therapy.

Anti-Inflammatory Agents

Both steroidal and nonsteroidal anti-inflammatory agents have been shown to be useful adjuncts. "Trigger point injections" might also facilitate physical therapy.

TENS

Transcutaneous electrical nerve stimulation (TENS) has unpredictable results, but is simple and non-invasive.

Antidepressants

This group has intrinsic analgesic effects, but does not cause tolerance or dependence.

There are no controlled studies which allow for evaluation of other therapies.

REFERENCES

1. Wilson, P.R. Sympathetically maintained pain: Diagnosis and therapy. In: Pain and the sympathetic nervous system (Stanton-Hicks, M.D.A. Editor. Kluwer Academic Publishers, Boston, 1989.

2. IASP Subcommittee on Taxonomy. Pain terms: A list with definitions and notes on usage. Pain, 6 (3): 249-252, 1979.

3. Raja, S.N., Meyer, R.A., Campbell, J.N. Peripheral mechanisms of somatic pain. Anesthesiology, 68: 571-590, 1988.

4. Devor, M. Central changes mediating neuropathic pain. In: Proceedings of the Vth World Congress on Pain (Dubner, R., Gebhart, G. F., Bond, M.R., eds.). Elsevier, Amsterdam, pp. 114-128, 1988.

5. Rowlingson, J.C. The sympathetic dystrophies. Int. Anesthesiol. Clin., 21: 117-129, 1983.

6. Schwartzman, R.J., McLellan, T.L. Reflex sympathetic dystrophy, a review. Arch Neurol., 44: 555-561, 1987.

7. Wall, P.D. Stability and instability of central pain mechanisms. In: Proceedings of the Vth World Congress on Pain (Dubner, R., Gebhart, G.F., Bond, M.R., eds.). Elsevier, Amsterdam, New York, Oxford, pp. 13-24, 1988.

8. Roberts, W.J. A hypothesis on the physiological basis for causalgia and related pains. Pain, 24: 297-311, 1986.

5

PSYCHOSOMATIC ASPECTS OF REFLEX SYMPATHETIC DYSTROPHY

U.T. Egle and S.O. Hoffmann

INTRODUCTION

Studies describing patients with reflex sympathetic dystrophy as neurotic, unbalanced and easily irritable have been published as early as the 1920s (1,2); similar statements continue to appear in studies published during the 1930s (3,4). The only pathogenetic concept, including an explicitly psychogenic component known to us, was developed by De Takats and Miller in 1943. These authors considered the patients' psychological status to be of vital importance to the autonomic reflexes, and therefore to the development of RSD (Sudeck-Syndrome). The patients are characterized as anxious and tense, exhibiting neuroautonomic stigmata, "inactive and hypertensive" (5). Langston and Covan (6) based their findings on the assumption of a clearly defined predisposed personality whose most pronounced characteristics are hypertension and a tense nervous system. Hübner (7) refers to the "Sudeck-personality" defining these patients as particularly sensitive, relatively detached, while simultaneously exhibiting a tendency to self-observation, and not infrequently an inclination to hypochondria. These observations were confirmed by an initial empirical investigation (8), subjecting twelve Sudeck-patients to psychological testing. Following evaluation of their results, the authors came to the conclusion that reflex sympathetic dystrophy presumably belongs to the group of actual psychosomatic disorders, whose principal pathogenetic aspect is determined by both premorbid psychological elements and somatic symptoms.

Most clinical researchers, however, felt that the reliability of the methods employed had not yet been confirmed, thus leaving the data open to question. A frequent argument was that the psychological disorders observed are not the cause, but rather the result of the chronic pain experienced (9).

EMPIRICAL INVESTIGATIONS

Most researchers arguing against the pathogenetic significance of psychogenic aspects were unaware of the more recent findings published by Zachariae (10). This investigator followed the postoperative course of one hundred patients with Dupuytren's contraction, who had undergone surgery in her clinic.   In forty-seven patients, an extensive psychiatric evaluation had been administered; on the basis of this evaluation an attempt was made to predict the postoperative clinical course of reflex sympathetic dystrophy.   The surgeon performing the operation was not aware of the outcome of the psychiatric evaluation.   The impressive result of this investigation is the correct prognostication of the postoperative clinical course in forty-three out of forty-seven cases.   (Table 1) In thirty-two patients, the prognosis of a clinical course without complications could be confirmed.   In ten patients, temporary complications of the clinical course had been prognosticated and actually occurred in eight of these cases, while the clinical course was not remarkable in the other two patients.   In five patients, severe complications of the clinical course had been prognosticated, and occurred in three of the cases while the clinical course in the remaining two patients was without complications.   Zachariae's results show that potential RSD patients are apparently characterized by aggressive inhibition, lack of self-assurance, self-absorption, self-pity, and hysterical personality traits.   Based on their investigation of forty patients with reflex sympathetic dystrophy following distal radius fracture, Pollack et al. (11) defined two different patient-types.   Using a personality inventory (Freiburg personality inventory) and an anxiety questionnaire (Spreen), the investigators were able to establish a basis for comparison with a control group exhibiting the same trauma.

TABLE 1. Preoperative Psyche in Relation to Postoperative Course

Psychiatric assessment	No. of cases	Presumed postop. course	Actual postop. course conformable	Actual postop. course not conformable
Normal	7	Uncomplicated	7	
Unstable	17	Uncomplicated	17	
Demented and arteriosclerotic	6	Uncomplicated	6	
Psychopathic	1	Uncomplicated	1	
Schizophrenic	1	Uncomplicated	1	
Aggression inhibited Defeatist attitude Self-pitying Perfectionistic Non-sthenic	10	Short-lasting difficulties in restitution	8	2
Aggression inhibited Martyr type Self-pitying Aggressive Self-opinionated Ambitious Hysterical Sthenic	5	Long-lasting severe complications	3	2
Total number	47		43	4

RESULTS

The following personality traits were observed in Type A patients:

a) increased anxiety reaction resulting in an over reaction to all internal and external stimuli as well as to the pain stimulus itself;

b) increased emotional instability characterized by undue reactions to outside events, most often focusing on the accident or surgery, accompanied by a high degree of nervousness and inability to act independently;

c) inclination to depressive reaction accompanied by pessimistic tendencies, feelings of inferiority, and insufficiency. In some cases, a tearful note in a patient's voice and the plaintive drift of his conversational topics provide an immediate indication of these tendencies;

d) psychosomatic disorders, e.g., intensive autonomic reactions following emotional experiences;

e) an over protective attitude toward the injured hand, which is frequently wrapped in a thick woolen cloth and steadied with the contralateral limb, although the arm usually is already in a sling. These patients are frequently accompanied by another person when they consult the treating therapist.

Type B patients constitute approximately one third of the patients participating in the study and Pollack et al. (11) observed the presence of the following personality traits in this group:

a) an exaggerated feeling of self-confidence, coupled with a strong need for communication and an obvious interest in social contacts;

b) a strong inclination to lying with a tendency toward dissimulation, an evasive attitude concerning critical self-examination, and the desire to present an attractive public image;

c) increased extroversion accompanied by impulsiveness and spontaneity.

A study published by DeLeo et al. (12), who administered the Eysenck Personality Inventory (MPI) to thirty-nine Sudeck-patients, confirmed Pollack's definition of Type A. Patients with reflex sympathetic dystrophy were observed to be significantly more introverted than patients of the control group.

An investigation of twenty-three 9 to 16 year-old children with reflex dystrophy revealed that prior to the onset of reflex dystrophy (13), this group showed high motivation in general, and was rated as highly achievement-directed in academic areas as well as in sports. After onset of the disease, most of the young patients were observed to be remarkably passive and indifferent concerning the restrictions imposed on their previous activities. The conspicuous absence of any demonstration of opposition or rebelliousness generally observed in young adolescents led the authors to the conclusion that the disease offered the children and adolescents a disguised possibility of aggressive confrontation with their parents. They were thus able to frustrate parental demands for performance and success without having to accept the responsibility for the disappointment caused, using the disease as justification for their low achievement. Ruggeri et al. (14) reached a similar conclusion in their investigation of children with reflex sympathetic dystrophy.

CLINICAL EXPERIENCE

Eight patients with RSD underwent an extensive clinical examination and comprehensive psychological testing at our clinic. An investigation of the patients' personal history showed that at the time of trauma or operation, and the subsequent onset of RSD, all patients were going through what was described as an extraordinarily difficult period in their lives. Surgical intervention therefore occurred at much the same time as an already existing life-crisis. The patients were unable to cope with this crisis and the narcissistic humiliation involved at the professional (e.g., demotion) or personal level (e.g., divorce). Five of the eight patients (all female) displayed the character traits attributed to Type A by Pollack et al. (11), while three patients (all male) were identified as Type B. An investigation of the patients' history during childhood and adolescence showed that four out of eight patients had spent the first years of life either in an orphanage or with foster parents, while the remaining four had experienced a difficult childhood according to criteria established by Engel (15) in his Pain-Proneness study.

To gain an understanding of the psychodynamics involved, we adopted the hypothesis put forward by Adler et al. (8) with regard to a narcissistic dynamic, i.e., the external and internal withdrawal resulting from a lack of self-confidence. External withdrawal is frequently observed following minor trauma, and is not uncommon with reflex sympathetic dystrophy.

The factor causing the disease and determining its clinical course is, therefore, not the intensity of the objective trauma, but a narcissistic reaction and subsequent depressive withdrawal marked by inertia and self-indulgence or unconsciously accusing/appealing behaviour ("look what you have done to me, now see what you get"). The imagined withdrawal from the outside world to the affected organ--a phenomenon also observed with hypochondria--may take a more depressive or more hysterical course in these patients, depending on the individual's basic personality.

The topic of psychodynamics leads to the subject of the disease as an equivalent to depression and its predominantly masochistic focus on suffering. This masochistic factor must be alluded to when statements like "patients assume the role of the martyr" or "the patient is making a cult of the disease" appear in clinical studies. Internal dynamics may furthermore offer the possibility of integrating reflex sympathetic dystrophy into the mainstream of the psychodynamics of chronic pain as was first attempted by Engel (15) and later impressively by Blumer and Heilbronn (16) as well as by Groen (17). A patient's social relationships and his objective relationships are of major importance, influencing the disposition for the disease as well as the clinical course. The somewhat limited results published on this subject (13) coincide with our observations in chronic pain patients: The influence of the attitude shown by the patient's relatives is of similar importance in RSD patients affecting both, length of the clinical course and the unconscious resort to the illness, in conflict situations arising in the family. In the course of these investigations, we have observed that each of the eight patients, tried to initiate confrontations between the different treating specialists, and four of the patients discontinued treatment following aggressive arguments with the treating clinician. These reactions again confirm extreme susceptibility and a basic narcissistic dynamic in these patients.

REFERENCES

1. Raeschke, H. Bemerkungen zum traumatischen chronischen Oedem. 1927.

2. Nippert, A. Konstitution, Stoffwechsel und Dupuytren'sche Kontraktur. 1955.

3. Orbach, E. Über die Pathogenese des sogenannten traumatischen Oedems. 1934.

4. de Takats, G. Reflex dystrophy of the extremities. Archs. Surgery, 34: 939-956, 1937; Post-traumatic dystrophy of the extremities. Archs. Surgery, 46: 469-479, 1943.

5. Moberg, E. The shoulder-hand-finger syndrome as a whole. Acta chir. Scandinavica, 109: 284-292, 1955.

6. Langston, R.G., Covan, R.J. Dupuytren's contracture. J. Internat. Coll. Surg., 23: 710, 1955.

7. Hübner, L. Das Sudeck-Syndrom. Der Landarzt, 3: 651-657, 1957.

8. Adler, E. A psychosomatic approach to sympathetic reflex dystrophie. Psychiat. Neurol., 138: 256-271, 1959.

9. Bonica, J.J. Causalgia and other reflex sympathetic dystrophies. In J.J. Bonica et al. (eds.), Advances in pain research and therapy. New York, 1979.

10. Zachariae, L. Incidence and course of posttraumatic dystrophy following operation for Dupuytren's contracture. Acta chir. Scand., Suppl. 336, 1964.

11. Pollack, H.-J., Neumann, R., Pollack, E. Morbus Sudeck und Psyche. Beitr. Orthopäd. Traumatol., 27: 463-468, 1980.

12. de Leo, D. Psychologische Faktoren beim Sudeck, Syndrom. DMW, 108: 719, 1982; Melzack, R., Wall, P.D. The challenge of pain. Basic Books, New York, 1982.

13. Bernstein, B.H., Singsen, B.H., Kent, J.T., Kornreich, H., King, K., Hicks, R., Hanson, V. Reflex neurovascular dystrophy in childhood. J. Pediatrics, 93: 211-215, 1978.

14. Ruggeri, S.B., Athereya, B.H., Doughty, R., Gregg, J.R., Das, M.M. Reflex sympathetic dystrophy in children. Clin. Orthopaed. Rel. Res., 163: 225-230, 1982.

15. Engel, G.L. "Psychogenic" pain and the pain-prone patient. Amer. J. Med., 26: 899-918, 1959.

16. Blumer, D., Heilbronn, M. Chronic pain as a variant of depressive disease. The pain-prone disorder. J. Nerv. Ment. Dis., 170: 381-406, 1982.

17. Groen, J.J.   Das Syndrom des sogenannten "unbehandelbaren Schmerzes." Psychother. Psychosom. Med. Psychol., 34: 27-32, 1984.

SUMMARY OF SECTION I

GENERAL CONSIDERATIONS

Much of the discussion centered around the imprecision of conventional diagnostic criteria and the heterogenous terminology that is used to describe symptoms and signs in patients described as having Reflex Sympathetic Dystrophy. The question of a diagnosis of RSD in the absence of any initiating event and the fact that some of the stigmata of RSD may present without any pain. It was obvious from the discussion that a proportionate increase in the number of patients presenting with contemporary criteria of RSD occurs as soon as attempts to develop diagnostic criteria are made.

It seems clear that no sex related differences occurred but that there was a peak incidence between the fifth and sixth decades. However, these differences may be a question of diagnostic criteria. An important observation made by Dr. Blumberg related to an apparent differential effect of the sympathetic activity on venules and arterioles, i.e., changing patterns of sympathetic on these two structures. Edema may or may not form as a result.

Patients presenting with RSD can be generally summarized into three groups: the first having autonomic disturbances, the second having motor disturbances and a constant fine tremor, and the third group has disturbances of sensation. Additionally, RSD is a disease which affects the entire distal extremity, irrespective of its source.

The group clearly felt that in addition to those accepted signs and symptoms including burning pain, hyperpathia/allodynia, temperature/color changes, edema and hair-nail growth that the most useful laboratory tests are thermography/thermometry and three phase bone scintigraphy. A sense developed in the course of the discussion that the response to a sympathetic block, while an adjunct to other diagnostic criteria, was more useful for reducing overall sympathetic activity, providing analgesia and facilitating rehabilitation.

Recent psychosomatic evidence has demonstrated an association between the development of Reflex Sympathetic Dystrophy and sympathetically mediated pain and the psychological personality of the patient. Such patients tend to be type A personalities.

Section II

BASIC RESEARCHES IN PATHOPHYSIOLOGY OF RSD

6

PATHOBIOLOGY OF REFLEX SYMPATHETIC DYSTROPHY: SOME GENERAL CONSIDERATIONS

Wilfrid Jänig
Supported by the Deutsche Forschungsgmeinschaft

INTRODUCTION

Under pathophysiological conditions, the sympathetic supply to the extremities may acquire a remarkable role in the generation and maintenance of pain states that are designated by the generic term *reflex sympathetic dystrophy* (RSD). Syndromes ranging under this general term appear to be extraordinarily variable and therefore have been described in the literature of the last 100 years under many names, indicating that the neuronal mechanisms are barely understood. Yet it is generally, though not unanimously, agreed that the (efferent) sympathetic nervous system is in some way or another involved in the generation of these pain syndromes.

This paper discusses the pathobiology of RSD, concentrating in particular on the role of the sympathetic nervous system. Some clinical key data will be described first, as least as they are seen from the experimental neurobiologist's point of view. On the basis of the clinical phenomenology, a general hypothesis about the pathophysiology of RSD will be formulated. Such a hypothesis cannot be expected to explain all clinical phenomena associated with RSD. It rather may serve to design experiments that enable investigation of the different components of RSD. On the basis of this more general hypothesis, some experimental data and specific ideas will be discussed.

CLINICAL DATA

The details of the clinical phenomenology, of the time course and of the therapy of RSD, as well as the events leading to it, are described extensively in the clinical contributions of this volume and in the literature (1,13,14). Table 1 illustrates a modified clinical subclassification of the RSD. This is a descriptive classification based on the intensity of symptoms, and does not imply different peripheral and central neural mechanisms. It has been introduced by Lücking and Blumberg (21) as a basis for diagnosis and therapy of RSD. The symptoms and clinical findings that establish the diagnosis RSD, are detailed by Wilson (Chapter 4), and include pain (burning, spontaneous, allodynia), disturbed regulation of cutaneous blood in the affected extremity (including disturbed thermoregulation), trophic changes of skin, appendages and subcutaneous tissue, and disturbances of active and passive motor performances including tremor.

TABLE 1. Three Proposed Subgroups of RSD

---

1) Sympathetic algodystrophy
   This group is the largest one; patients with sympathetic algodystrophy have all symptoms.

2) Sympathetic dystrophy
   Patients with this phenomenology do not have the typical burning pain, but evidence all other symptoms.

3) Sympathetic maintained pain
   These patients have typical spontaneous pain and allodynia, but no obvious disturbance of regulation of blood flow, no obvious trophic changes and only discrete motor disturbances. It is not easy to recognize this type of RSD; therefore it may be misdiagnosed.

An important reason to use the generic term reflex sympathetic dystrophy (RSD) is the experience that temporary or permanent blockade of sympathetic activity to the affected extremity, by whatever means, commonly (but not always) relieves or abolishes the pain. When sustained, this is followed by a restitution of the trophic changes and of the disturbed autonomic regulation, provided this procedure has been performed early enough (1,4,11,23,24,28). This frequently applied therapeutic procedure clearly indicates that the sympathetic nervous system is involved in the generation of RSD. It does not indicate in which way that occurs.

Different classes of events that may induce RSD indicate that peripheral (neural and non-neural) and central mechanisms are involved:

I. Most common and probably most important are <u>mechanical traumata</u> at the extremities that include peripheral nerves (19,24,25,27,29). The lesion of nerves is not always obvious, particularly when soft tissues of an extremity are traumatized. Causalgias as the rare extremes of RSD are mostly associated with traumata of proximal nerves such as the sciatic nerve, the median nerve and the cervico-brachial plexus (26,27). The typical nerve lesion in causalgia is not a complete one but a partial one, that leaves many nerve fibers intact. RSD may also develop after trivial nerve and other peripheral traumata.

II. <u>Excitation of spinal visceral afferents</u> under pathophysiological condition (e.g., by angina pectoris and heart infarction) (8,15,28).

III. <u>Lesions in the central nervous system</u> such as in the thalamus, the brain stem and the spinal cord without direct involvement of peripheral nerves (15,21, 22,25,30).

The latter two "causes" are rare, yet probably important and interesting, for understanding of the mechanism of RSD.

HYPOTHESIS ABOUT THE GENERATION OF REFLEX SYMPATHETIC DYSTROPHY

Figure 1 presents in schematic form a general hypothesis on the pathophysiological mechanisms of RSD. The main clinical phenomena (Table 1) are put in double-framed boxes. The events that may lead to RSD are put at the top of the figure in simple boxes. The diagram has a heuristic character, putting apparently unrelated phenomena together. Some components of this diagram are not new and have already been described by Livingston (19) and others (1,2,11,14). Several peripheral and central processes seem to interact

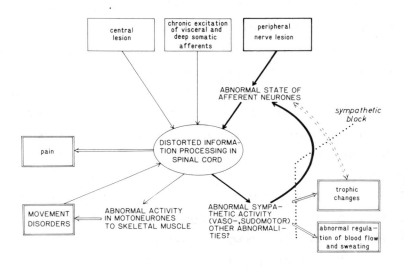

Fig. 1
General hypothesis about the neural mechanisms of generation of RSD following peripheral nerve lesions, central lesions and chronic stimulation of visceral afferents. Note the vicious circle (arrows in black). An important component of this circle is the excitatory influence of postganglionic sympathetic axons on primary afferent fibers in the periphery. This influence leads to orthodromic afferent impulse activity. But it may also induce antidromically conducted impulses in unmyelinated afferents to the periphery which may contribute to the trophic changes (i.e., by release of substances due to antidromic invasion of axon terminals which leads to vasodilation and plasma extravasation). These trophic changes may in turn influence the coupling between postganglionic axons and afferent axons (see interrupted double arrow). Another important component not emphasized in this diagram may be that the neurovascular transmission is impaired and that the blood vessels develop adaptive supersensitivity to changes in the local micromilieu (e.g., to released vasoactive substances), to circulating substances, to external influences (e.g., increase and decrease of environmental temperatures) and to nerve impulses. For details see text. Modified from (1,14).

with each other, and the quantitative predominance of one or the other process may determine the diversity of the clinical phenomenology, its time course and its response to different therapies.

1) The main component of the hypothesis is a change of the processing of the information in the spinal cord and possibly in supraspinal brain centers. This change is reflected in the following features:

I. Abnormal pain.

II. Abnormal sympathetic activity. This follows from the abnormal neuronal regulation of skin blood flow and sweat secretion. The trophic changes are possibly also--at least in part--a consequence of the abnormal sympathetic activity.

III. Abnormal motor activity. The resting tremor changes, and active and passive movements are disturbed.

2) Another component in the generation of RSD is probably the coupling between sympathetic postganglionic axons and afferent axons in the periphery which establishes a *vicious circle* (heavily drawn arrows Fig. 1). This circle may maintain the pathophysiological process which is interrupted by sympathetic blocks (dotted line, Fig. 1).

3) The peripheral pathophysiological coupling between postganglionic and afferent axons may not only lead to orthodromic afferent impulse activity to the spinal cord, but also to antidromic afferent activity to the periphery. Antidromic activity in unmyelinated afferents may initiate the "axon response" (vasodilation and plasma extravasation) in peripheral tissues (6,16,17). This may contribute to the abnormal regulation of the blood flow and the trophic changes in the peripheral tissues and to changes in micromilieu of the afferent receptors (interrupted double line with arrows).

4) Blood vessels and other autonomic effector organs develop adaptive supersensitivity to circulating catecholamines and other substances after degeneration of their innervation (9). This component is rarely taken into account and has barely been investigated. For instance it is not known (though

tacitly accepted), whether blood vessels are fully reinnervated by noradrenergic vasoconstrictor fibers and unmyelinated afferent fibers after degeneration, or whether they then exhibit abnormal reactions to normal sympathetic activity.

5) Central lesions and pathophysiological stimulation of visceral afferents (e.g., in angina pectoris) may produce the symptomatology of RSD (8,15,20, 22,28). It is hypothesized that central lesions change the descending control systems of the spinal circuits and that long lasting intense abnormal activity in visceral afferents lead to changes of the spinal information processing with the same consequences as observed after nerve lesions.

EXPERIMENTAL DATA SUPPORTING THE HYPOTHESIS

The hypothesis, as outlined above, cannot be proven as such, offering a heuristic rather than a scientific hypothesis that can be tested experimentally. Many components of this hypothesis can, however, be supported by experimental data.

The changes that may take place after peripheral nerve lesions at the level of the primary afferent neuron and the sympathetic postganglionic neuron, at the spinal cord and supraspinal levels, and at target organs are listed in Table 2. It is not conditional for the development of RSD that these changes occur together. However, it is rather crucial to understand that the diversity of these neurobiological changes that could occur, may explain the remarkable variability of the clinical features described in the preceding chapters. They may also explain why one or other symptom dominates the clinical picture, and that there is not a single mechanism which generates RSD. Similarly, these features may explain why unimodal therapy can be ineffective. Peripheral and central mechanisms that may contribute to the generation of RSD after mechanical peripheral nerve lesions. Some of these mechanisms may also contribute to the generation of RSD after peripheral trauma without (obvious) nerve lesion, after chronic excitation of visceral afferents and after central lesions. Some of these processes have been worked out in neurobiological experiments and are well established. Some are speculative and hypothetical (modified after (14); see 11-13); for literature see same).

TABLE 2.

A. <u>Primary afferent neuron, postganglionic sympathetic neuron</u>

1. Retrograde cell reactions: biochemical changes as expression of repair involving neurons in their entirety; decrease in neuropeptide content in primary afferent neurons; atrophy and degeneration of neurons
2. Anterograde cell reactions: sprouting of fibers with axon-receptor and postganglionic-target organ mismatch; neuroma formation
3. Development of abnormal membrane properties of afferent sprouts: generation of resting activity, abnormal chemosensitivity (e.g., to noradrenalin) and mechanosensitivity of sprouting afferent neurons
4. Changes of receptive properties of intact primary afferent fibers by change of micromilieu (ischemia, release of sensitizing and vasoactive substances); sensitizing of afferent receptors
5. Development of ephaptic transmission among afferent fibers in the lesioned territory and nerve, this being possibly an amplifier for afferent activity
6. Development of "cross-talk" between postganglionic sympathetic fibers and afferent fibers: chemical (by release of noradrenalin), ephaptic (unlikely), indirectly by change of micromilieu
7. Change and failure of synaptic transmission from preganglionic to postganglionic neurons in sympathetic ganglia and from primary afferent neurons on dorsal horn neurons

B. <u>Spinal cord</u>

1. Changes in distribution of primary afferent axon terminals in the spinal cord (degeneration, sprouting)
2. Unmasking of synapses from primary afferents on second order neurons; formation of new aberrant synaptic connections
3. Biochemical changes in dorsal horn neurons (e.g., decrease of peptide content); development of supersensitivity to neurotransmitters and neuromodulators due to deafferentation
4. Change of inhibitory control mechanisms in the dorsal horn (local and descending from the brain stem); change of receptive fields and discharge properties of dorsal horn neurons; change of somatotopic map
5. Development of abnormal discharge properties and abnormal reflexes in sympathetic neurons supplying the affected extremity (skin, deep somatic tissue etc.)

TABLE 2. (continued)

---

6.   Development of abnormal discharge properties and abnormal reflexes in motoneurons supplying the affected extremity

C.   Target organs

1.   Development of adaptive supersensitivity and sub-sensitivity of autonomic effector organs on degeneration and regeneration of their neural supply; abnormal responses to neural impulses, substances released locally, circulating substances and external influences (e.g., changes in environmental temperature)

2.   Abnormal regulation of blood flow through skin and subcutaneous tissues; mismatch of vasoconstrictor activity to different sections of vascular beds

3.   Increase of filtration pressure in capillary beds with subsequent chronic formation of edemata due to imbalance of pre- to postcapillary constriction; increase in vascular permeability due to release of vasoactive substances (e.g., from primary afferents or local cells) or due to other processes

4.   Atrophy and degeneration of dermis, capillaries, subcutis, joint capsules; rarification of bones, etc.

---

1) For the development of *pain*, one or several abnormalities might appear in the nociceptive and other somatosensory pathways. This may happen at the level of the primary afferent neuron (changes of receptors, atopic impulse generators of lesioned axons) in the spinal cord (changes in synaptic transmission, changes in inhibitory local and descending control mechanisms etc.), and in supraspinal brain centers. It must always be kept in mind that these changes take time in order to develop; so does the recovery. Furthermore, it must be kept in mind that they occur on the basis of considerable biomechanical changes that are then seen in an altered morphology. For instance, degeneration and death of neurons and changes of intraneural transport processes that are probably important signals in the reciprocal communication between spinal cord and target organs. It is conceivable that the chronic pain may also appear when the central nociceptive system gets into disorder after central lesions, or when it is continuously "bombarded" by impulse

activity in spinal visceral afferents from internal organs and possibly in small diameter afferents from deep somatic structures.

2) Changes in the central nociceptive and possibly other somatosensory neural processes, comprise also changes in the motor output system of the spinal cord, namely the *motoneurons* to the skeletal muscle and the *sympathetic system* to skin and subcutaneous tissues. Passive and active motor disorders, while reported in the literature, are not well understood (in particular, the sometimes beneficial effect of sympathetic blocks) and have not been systematically investigated. Neither is the abnormal regulation of blood flow (and sometimes sweating) understood, even though they may be leading symptoms in the diagnosis of RSD. The reflex patterns in cutaneous vasoconstrictor neurons to adequate afferent stimuli may dramatically change a long time after an experimental nerve lesion has been performed at one of the extremities (3).

3) The abnormal sympathetic activity is probably also related to the *trophic changes* that are seen in skin, skin appendages (nails and hairs), and subcutaneous tissues (subcutis, bone, joint capsules, etc); these changes may disappear after blockade of the sympathetic activity. It seems as if the first sign of trophic changes is edema, that might be produced by functional abnormalities in the sympathetic (and afferent) supply of the microvascular bed (13). Again, it must not be forgotten that sympathetic and afferent neurons do not only conduct impulses, but are also transport systems of materials, and that both types of neurons may be involved in local regulation, release of substances, etc.

4) A crucial component of the mechanisms of RSD appears to be the *coupling between postganglionic sympathetic and afferent axons*. Theoretically this coupling could occur in several ways (12,13). There is ample experimental evidence for chemical coupling (by release of noradrenalin) (2,7,10). Other ways of coupling (e.g., by ephapses, indirectly by changes of the micromilieu of the primary afferent fibers), however, should not be discarded.

5) A component that has been very much neglected is the effect of the *afferent and sympathetic innervation of blood vessels* in the territory of the lesioned nerves. What are the mechanisms of adaptive supersensitivity (after denervation) and subsensitivity of blood vessels? (9) To what extent does the regulation of the circulation in skin and subcutaneous tissues depend on activity in small diameter afferents? In this context, the axon response ("axon reflex") (6,18) may come into the "game." Does the influence of activity in fine diameter afferents on blood vessels interact with the activity in sympathetic postganglionic vaso-constrictor neurons? Is the neural regulation of blood vessels impaired after regeneration of their innervation and during changes of the micromilieu of the lesioned and adjacent territories? Does there exist an imbalance between the effects of neural signals and non-neural signals (e.g., locally released vasoactive substances, circulating substances) on the blood vessels? These questions have barely been studied.

SUMMARY

The spinal cord is not a brain center that mediates afferent information in a relay-like fashion from the periphery to ascending systems, motoneurons and sympathetic neurons. It contains many "neural programs" that "recognize" the information from the periphery, and channel it to these output systems. All three exhibit changes with long-term changes of the afferent inputs. Spinal and supraspinal neuronal processes may generate abnormal patterns of activity with partial or complete deafferentation (e.g., after peripheral nerve lesions) or with central lesions or even with a persistent afferent inflow to the spinal cord from diseased internal organs and deep somatic tissues, leading to distorted sensory phenomena (paresthesias, neurogenic pains), skeletomotor reactions and autonomic reactions. In the periphery the autonomic effector organs may change too, and develop adaptive supersensitivity and subsensitivity to circulating substances, nerve impulses and changes in the local milieu. Thus, the abnormal afferent messenges impinge on a central neuronal system that is also changed as a consequence of the peripheral nerve injury; this in turn may be reflected in abnormal sympathetic activity that again meets a target organ in the periphery which is changed too. The multiple interacting peripheral and central changes that may occur in the nociceptive system, in the skeletomotor system and the sympathetic systems, as a consequence of the peripheral and central lesions and abnormal afferent activities, generate a syndrome in patients that is described by the generic term "reflex sympathetic dystrophy." In many cases the sympathetic activity to the affected extremity may be crucial in the generation of this syndrome. This, however, probably does not apply to all cases of RSD.

REFERENCES

1. Blumberg, H., Jänig, W. Changes of reflexes in vasoconstrictor neurons supplying the cat hindlimb following chronic nerve lesions: a model for studying mechanisms of reflex sympathetic dystrophy? J. Auton. Nerv. Syst., 7: 399-411, 1983.

2. Blumberg, H., Jänig, W. Discharge pattern of afferent fibers from a neuroma. Pain, 20: 335-353, 1984.

3. Blumberg, H., Jänig, W. Reflex patterns and post ganglionic vasoconstrictor neurons following chronic nerve lesions. J. Auton. Nerv. Syst., 14: 157-180, 1985.

4. Bonica, J.J. (1953) The management of pain. Lea and Febiger, Philadelphia; reprinted by Honji Shoji Company, Tokyo, 1980.

5. Bonica, J.J. Causalgia and other reflex sympathetic dystrophies. In J.J. Bonica, J.C. Liebeskind, D.G. Albe-Fessard (Eds.), Advances in Pain Research and Therapy, Vol. 3. Raven Press, New York, pp. 141-166, 1979.

6. Chahl, L.A., Szolcsányi, J., Lembeck, F. (eds.). Antidromic vasodilatation and neurogenic inflammation (1984). Akademiai Kiado, Budapest.

7. Devor, M., Jänig, W. Activation of myelinated afferents ending in a neuroma by stimulation of the sympathetic supply in the rat. Neurosci. Lett., 24: 43-47, 1981.

8. Doury, P., Dirheimer, Y., Pattin, S. Algodystrophy. Springer, Berlin, Heidelberg, New York, 1981.

9. Fleming,   W.W.,   Westfall,   D.P.   Adaptive   supersensitivity.   In Trendelenburg, U. and Weiner, N. (eds.) Catecholamines I. Handbook of Experimental Pharmacology. Vol 90/I, Springer-Verlag, Berlin Heidelberg, pp. 509-559, 1988.

10. Häbler, H.-J., Jänig, W., Koltzenburg, M. Activation of unmyelinated afferents in chronically lesioned nerves by adrenaline and excitation of sympathetic afferents in the cat. Neurosci. Lett., 82: 35-40, 1987.

11. Jänig, W. Causalgia and reflex sympathetic dystrophy: In which way is the sympathetic nervous system involved? Trends in Neurosci., 8: 471-477, 1987.

12. Jänig, W. Pathophysiology of nerve following mechanical injury. In R. Dubner, G.F. Gebhart, M.R. Bond (Eds.), Proceedings of the Vth World Congress on Pain. Pain Research and Clinical Management. Vol. 3, Elsevier Science Publishers, Amsterdam, pp. 89-108, 1988.

13. Jänig, W. The sympathetic nervous system in pain: physiology and pathophysiology. In Stanton-Hicks (ed.), "Sympathetic Nervous System and Pain," in press. (1989)

14. Jänig, W., Kollmann, W. The involvement of the sympathetic nervous system in pain. Arzneim.- Forsch./Drug Res., 34 (II): 1066-1073, 1984.

15. Kozin, F., Ryan, L.M., Carrera, G.F., Soin, J.S., Wortmann, R.L. The reflex sympathetic dystrophy syndrome (RSDS). III. Scintigraphic studies, further evidence for the therapeutic efficacy of systemic corticosteroids, and proposed diagnostic criteria. Amer. J. Med., 70: 23-30, 1981.

16. Lembeck, F. Sir Thomas Lewis's nocifensor system, histamine and substance-P-containing primary afferent nerves. Trends in Neuroscience,

6: 106-108, 1983.

17. Lewis, T. Pain. The Macmillan Press LTD, 1982.

18. Lisney, S.J.W., Bharali, L.A.M. The axon reflex. Is it an outdated idea or still a valid hypothesis? Trends in Physiological Sciences, in press. (1989)

19. Livingston, W.K. Pain mechanisms. A physiologic interpretation of causalgia and its related states. Plenum Press, New York, London. Reprint of the 1943 ed. published by Macmillan, New York, 1976.

20. Loh, L., Nathan, P.W., Schott, G.D. Pain due to lesions of central nervous system removed by sympathetic block. Brit. Med. J., 282: 1026-1028, 1981.

21. Lücking, C.H., Blumberg, H., Kausalgie und sympathische Reflexdystrophie, Fischer Verlag, 1988.

22. Moskowitz, E., Bishop, H.F., Pe, H., Shibutani, K. Posthemiplegic reflex sympathetic dystrophy. I.A.M.A., 167: 836-838, 1958.

23. Payne, R. Neuropathic pain syndromes, with special reference to causalgia and reflex sympathetic dystrophy. The Clinical J. of Pain, 2: 59-73, 1986.

24. Richards, R.L. Causalgia. Arch. Neurol. 16: 339350, 1967.

25. Schott, G.D. Mechanisms of causalgia and related clinical conditions. The role of the central and of the sympathetic nervous system. Brain, 109: 717-738, 1986.

26. Sunderland, S. Pain mechanisms in causalgia. J. Neurol. Neurosurg. Psychiat., 39: 471-480, 1976.

27. Sunderland, S. Nerves and nerve injuries, 2nd ed., Churchill Livingstone, Edinburgh London New York, 1978.

28. Sweet, W.H., Poletti, C.E. Causalgia and sympathetic dystrophy (Sudeck atrophy). In G.M. Aronoff (Ed.), Evaluation and Treatment of Chronic Pain. Urban and Schwarzenberg, Baltimore Munchen, pp. 149-165, 1985.

29. Thorban, W. Das Sudeck'sche Syndrom. In A. Sturm, W. Birkmayer (eds.), Klinische Pathologie des vegetativen Nervensystems, Vol. 2. Gustav Fischer, Stuttgart, pp. 1186-1206, 1977.

30. Wainapel, S.F. Reflex sympathetic dystrophy following traumatic myelopathy. Pain, 18:345-349, 1984.

7

SPINAL HYPEREXCITABILITY IN SYMPATHETICALLY MAINTAINED PAIN

William J. Roberts

Anesthetic block of sympathetic postganglionic neurons relieves both spontaneous pain and mechanical allodynia in some individuals without blocking painful responses to noxious stimuli. A similar effect is obtained in many cases by regional infusion of guanethidine, which depletes norepinephrine from peripheral tissues. These responses to sympathetic block indicate that the pain and allodynia are *sympathetically maintained*--that they are dependent on sympathetic efferent activity. One syndrome characterized by sympathetically maintained pain is reflex sympathetic dystrophy.

The physiological basis for sympathetically maintained pain has long been assumed to be sympathetic efferent activation of primary afferent nociceptors. Sympathetic activation of nociceptors has been assumed to occur either at sensory receptors in the painful area (e.g., through ischemia) or intraneurally at a site of peripheral nerve damage (1).

However, attempts to demonstrate sympathetic activation of primary afferent nociceptors in experimental animals have been largely unsuccessful (2,3,4,) except for some myelinated nociceptors in intact nerves (5) and nonmyelinated afferents (possible nociceptors) associated neuromatin-continuity (6). Thus, the results from physiological studies to date provide little support for the hypothesis that sympathetic activation of primary afferent nociceptors is responsible for the pain and allodynia in these disorders.

The assumption that activity in *nociceptors* was responsible for the spontaneous pain and allodynia in disorders relieved by sympathetic block was challenged by Loh and Nathan (7), who suggested that *low-threshold mechanoreceptors*, not nociceptors, are responsible for the pain and allodynia. They suggested that mechanoreceptor activity resulted in pain because central pain pathways are hyperexcitable in these disorders (8).

The idea that activity in low-threshold mechanoreceptors can elicit pain is supported by the knowledge that some spinal sensory neurons receive convergent excitatory input from both low- and high-threshold primary afferents; these are the wide-dynamic-range or convergent neurons (9). These neurons show increased responses to afferent activity following brief noxious stimuli and are widely thought to be part of the spinal "pain" pathway.

This concept, that low-threshold mechanoreceptors might mediate sympathetically maintained pain, was tested physiologically with recordings of responses in low-threshold primary afferents to sympathetic stimulation. The results showed that some afferents in several classes of low-threshold mechanoreceptors are sympathetically activated (10).

This experimental support of Loh and Nathan's proposal led to formulation of the following hypothesis (10).

1) A precipitating trauma leads to sensitization of spinal wide-dynamic-range (WDR or convergent) neurons.

2) Subsequent sympathetic activation of low-threshold mechanoreceptors results in excessive firing of hyper excitable WDR neurons and therefore "spontaneous" pain.

3) Mechanical activation of low-threshold mechanoreceptors results in excessive firing of hyperexcitable WDR neurons and therefore pain (allodynia).

The essential dysfunction proposed in this hypothesis is hyperexcitability of spinal wide-dynamic-range neurons, not abnormal activation of nociceptors in the periphery.

Recent investigations of spinal neurons support this hypothesis (11,12). Recordings from single dorsal horn neurons show that many WDR neurons are activated by electrical stimulation of sympathetic efferent fibers in anesthetized cats. This activation is blocked by cooling of the receptive field or by alpha-adrenergic blockers, indicating that a peripheral, adrenergic mechanism provides the coupling between sympathetic efferent and primary afferent fibers.

The same investigations showed that nociceptor specific spinal neurons, which receive primary afferent input predominantly from nociceptors, are not activated by sympathetic stimulation. This result is consistent with the results of studies of sympathetic actions on primary afferent nociceptors (see above). This result also suggests that nociceptor-specific spinal neurons are not likely to mediate sympathetically maintained pain unless this class of neurons is much more responsive in patients than in anesthetized animals.

Ongoing studies of spinal neurons in our laboratory also indicate that brief noxious pinching or burning of the receptive field results in prolonged increases in responding to WDR neurons to sympathetic stimulation (unpublished observations). This finding provides additional support for the hypothesis that responses of WDR neurons to sympathetically evoked afferent activity are enhanced following noxious input.

Recent studies of patients with sympathetically maintained pain have provided additional evidence that low-threshold afferents mediate the spontaneous pain and allodynia in reflex sympathetic dystrophy. In these studies, pressure is applied to a limb to progressively block conduction in nerves that innervate a painful area. As expected, the sense of touch is lost first as the largest A-beta afferents are blocked. In patients with sympathetically maintained pain, *pressure block of only A-beta fibers also abolishes the spontaneous pain and mechanical allodynia* (13,14; Ochoa, Roberts, Cline, and Dotson, unpublished observations). This abolition of pain and allodynia occurs when pinprick, cold and warm stimuli are still perceived normally, indicating that A-delta and C-fibers are functional.

This clinical finding provides strong support for the hypothesis that sympathetically maintained pain is mediated by low-threshold mechanoreceptors.

The abolition of mechanical allodynia during sympathetic block is most likely explained as a disfacilitation of spinal wide-dynamic-range neurons. Block of sympathetic efferent activity presumably reduces tonic activity of low-threshold mechanoreceptors. This presumed reduction of afferent input reduces the excitatory drive on WDR neurons, making them respond at lower (non-painful) rates to non-noxious stimuli.

This physiological explanation for sympathetically maintained pain does not exclude the possibility that other mechanisms may simultaneously contribute to pain and allodynia. For example, sympathetic activation of primary afferents ending in a neuroma may contribute to the excitation of WDR neurons and sensitized nociceptors may also participate. In patients with complex disorders, it is not unlikely that several pathological processes are involved in the genesis of pain.

More physiological studies are needed to understand the spinal mechanisms that underlie the hyper excitability in these syndromes.

With present knowledge of physiological mechanisms, the best approach for preventing sympathetically maintained pain appears to be suppression of nociceptor input to the spinal cord. This might be done with regional or spinal anesthetic blocks, cooling of the nociceptors in an injured area, or anti-inflammatory agents. Most clinical reports also stress the value of repeated sympathetic blocks early in the development of this type of disorder.

REFERENCES

1. Jänig, W. Causalgia and reflex sympathetic dystrophy: In which way is the sympathetic nervous system involved? Trends in Neuroscience, 89: 471-477, 1985.

2. Roberts, W.J., Lindsay, A.D. Sympathetic activity shown to have no short-term effect on polymodal nociceptors in cats. Society for Neuroscience Abstracts, 7: 227, 1973.

3. Shea, V.K., Perl, E.R. Failure of sympathetic stimulation to effect responsiveness of rabbit polymodal nociceptors. J. of Neurophysiology, 54: 513-520, 1985.

4. Barasi, S., Lynn, B. Effects of sympathetic stimulation on mechanoreceptive and nociceptive afferent units from the rabbit pinna. Brain Res., 378: 21-27, 1986.

5. Roberts, W.J., Elardo, S.M. Sympathetic activation of A-delta nociceptors. Somatosensory Res., 3: 33-44, 1985.

6. Häbler, H.J., Jänig, W., Koltzenburg, M. Activation of unmyelinated afferents in chronically lesioned nerves by adrenalin and excitation of sympathetic efferents in the cat. Neuroscience Letters, 82: 35-40, 1987.

7. Loh, L., Nathan, P. W. Painful peripheral states and sympathetic blocks. J. Neurol. Neurosurg. Psychiat., 41: 664-671, 1978.

8. Wiesenfeld-Hallin, Z., Hallin, R.G. The influence of the sympathetic system on mechanoreception and nociception. A review. Human Neurobiology, 3: 41-46, 1984.

9. Besson, J.M., Chaouch, A. Peripheral and spinal mechanisms of nociception. Physiol. Rev., 67: 67-153, 1987.

10. Roberts, W.J. A hypothesis on the physiological basis for causalgia and related pains. Pain, 24: 297-311, 1986.

11. Roberts, W.J., Foglesong, M.E. I. Spinal recordings indicate that wide-dynamic-range neurons mediate sympathetically maintained pain. Pain, 34: 289-304, 1988.

12. Roberts, W.J., Foglesong, M.E. II. Identification of afferents contributing to sympathetically evoked activity in wide-dynamic-range neurons. Pain, 34: 305-314, 1988.

13. Campbell, J.N., Raja, S.N., Meyer, R.A., Mackinnon, S.E. Myelinated afferents signal the hyperalgesia associated with nerve injury. Pain, 32: 89-94, 1988.

14. Price, D.D., Bennett, G.J., Rafii, A. Psycho-physical observations on patients with neuropathic pain relieved by a sympathetic block. Pain (in press).

8

NEUROPHARMACOLOGICAL ASPECTS OF REFLEX SYMPATHETIC DYSTROPHY

Ilmar Jurna

Neuropharmacological studies on reflex sympathetic dystrophy started when it was first demonstrated (45), that adrenaline and noradrenaline excited afferent nerve fibres from experimental neuromas. Activation resulted from local application or systemic administration of the catecholamines.

Ectopic adrenoceptors

Wall and Gutnick also made an attempt to characterize the type of receptor involved. They found that the alpha-adrenoceptor antagonist phentolamine did not change activity in afferents from neuromas discharging spontaneously, but prevented activation by adrenaline or noradrenaline. Since, in addition, the beta-adrenoceptor agonist isoprenaline failed to activate the afferents, it was concluded that stimulation by both adrenaline and noradrenaline follows from binding to alpha receptors. These results have been confirmed in the following years by experiments in which it was observed that activity in afferents from experimental neuromas, was elicited or increased by local or systemic adrenaline or noradrenaline and the alpha-adrenoceptor agonist phenylephrine (27,36). This stimulant effect was also blocked by the alpha antagonist phentolamine, while the beta agonist isoprenaline produced no activation, and catecholamine-induced activation was not prevented by pretreatment with propranolol (27). Characterization of the adrenoceptor subtype responsible for the excitatory effect of adrenaline or noradrenaline by using the differential adrenoceptor ligands WB 4101 and clonidine, was not successful (8). Since unlesioned afferent nerve fibers do not respond to adrenaline or noradrenaline, it has been proposed that ectopic alpha-adrenoceptor binding sites either have newly formed receptors on afferents from the neuromas, or are an accumulation of receptors normally occurring on afferent fibers (8,27).

Sympathetic output

Activation of sympathetic efferents by electrical stimulation of preganglionic nerve fibers (10) or the spinal cord (27), also excited afferents from experimental neuromas. Although noradrenaline accumulates in the proximal endings of lesioned sympathetic axons (15,28), no noradrenergic terminals or synapses have been detected in neuromas (7). It has been suggested therefore that noradrenaline released from terminals of unlesioned sympathetic efferents reaches ectopic alpha-receptors on afferent lesioned nerves or sprouts, by penetration in the region of the neuroma or blood circulation. This in turn, produces a local depolarization generating repetitive discharges in the afferents (7). Although ischemia increased activity in afferents from neuromas, catecholamine induced excitation was not secondary to reduced blood circulation in the region (27).

Central events

Activity set up by noradrenaline (or adrenaline) in afferents from neuromas produce reflex activation of sympathetic efferents so that afferent activity is further increased and a vicious circle builds up (21). Inhibition by noxious stimulation of sympathetic output to the skin disappears after chronic nerve lesions so that the sympathetic output is increased (2). In addition to activity arising in lesioned afferents, activity is also generated in dorsal root ganglia of these afferents (6,24,42), which contributes to the impulse input entering the spinal cord. Moreover, processing of afferent signals in the spinal cord is markedly changed after having produced chronic lesions of nerves (41). Nerve section results in reorganization of synaptic contacts in the spinal cord, many deafferented neurones in the dorsal horn exhibiting a new receptive field (11,12,19,30). These changes disappear when regeneration occurs (12,31).

From this it may be expected that nociceptive activity is set up in ascending pathways so that pain is perceived. Pain behavior is induced by stress due to cold exposure in rats in which one limb was denervated (48). Most likely, these animals would have exhibited elevated plasma levels of adrenaline and noradrenaline. Autotomy of chronically denervated limbs in rats and mice is regarded as a model of anesthesia dolorosa (43).

APPROACHES TO PHARMACOTHERAPY

Sympathetic block

The central mechanisms underlying the symptoms of reflex sympathetic dystrophy have not yet been fully elucidated, but is evident that processes in the periphery are necessary to start or maintain the events causing the symptoms and offer the only rational basis for pharmacotherapy actually existing. The target is mostly the sympathetic system whose role, as outlined above, is further stressed by the observation that sympathetic block with local anesthetic agents or sympathectomy alleviates pain in patients (1,4,33,37,46). Failure of sympathectomy to produce lasting relief from pain in some, has been attributed to crossing of sympathetic nerve fibers (25). However, it is more likely that ectopic receptor sensitivity to circulating noradrenaline increases, in a similar way as the sensitivity to noradrenaline of sympathetically innervated organs increases after degeneration of the sympathetic nerves (14,20,29,32,40).

Guanethidine

Regional intravenous administration of guanethidine gives relief from pain in RSD as presented in Chapter 12 (16,17,33). Guanethidine also prevents autotomy of the denervated limb in rats and mice (44). Again, these effects are due to block of sympathetic nerve function, because guanethidine blocks the release of noradrenaline from sympathetic nerve terminals (47).

Neuroleptic agents

A beneficial effect may also be expected from neuroleptic agents. This is not necessarily due to an action on an as yet unknown central mechanism of reflex sympathetic dystrophy, but because neuroleptic agents are known to block peripheral adrenoceptors (13,22,34,35).

Interference with ion mechanisms

Apart from blocking sympathetic nerve function, interference with ion mechanisms in the membrane of lesioned nerve fibers might be useful in treating the symptoms resulting from nerve lesions. It has recently been shown that Phenytoin, applied systemically or topically to desheathed neuromas suppressed the generation of impulses in the afferents without blocking impulse conduction (49). Phenytoin may cause pain relief in neuralgias with shooting pain (38). Like the antiepileptic action of the drug, this effect is attributed to reduced conduction of sodium and calcium ions in the membranes of excitable tissues (23,38). It is interesting to note in this context that tetra-ethylammonium (TEA), which blocks potassium channels (18,26), was found to increase spontaneous impulse discharge in active afferents from experimental neuromas (3). On account of this result it was suggested that potassium conductance is elevated in afferents from neuromas which, in turn, reduces the tendency towards hyperexcitability and spontaneous impulse discharges.

Topical application of vinblastine and related alkaloids has been reported to reduce cutaneous hyperalgesia in patients (5). It is in accord with these observations that colchicine or vinblastine, which block axoplasmatic transport, applied to the proximal part of a nerve at the time of cutting the nerve, reduced spontaneous and adrenaline-induced activity in afferents from the neuroma (8). These effects were explained by prevention of the incorporation of sodium and calcium channels and of ectopic adrenoceptors into the membrane of sprouts and afferent nerve fibres.

Finally, the development of activity in afferents from neuromas is prevented when the freshly cut nerve end is treated with corticosteroids, and ongoing activity is depressed when corticosteroids are locally applied to neuromas (9). These effects were interpreted in terms of a direct action of corticosteroids on the membrane conductance of ions.

CONCLUSION

Reflex sympathetic dystrophy is a term that summarizes a syndrome resulting from various causes. Since at present only one experimental model exists which obviously cannot be representative for all causes, it is not surprising that a considerable number of patients suffering from reflex sympathetic dystrophy still awaits appropriate treatment with drugs.

REFERENCES

1. Betcher, A.M., Bean. G., Casten, D.F. Continuous procaine block of paravertebral sympathetic ganglions. Observations on one hundred patients. J. Am. Med. Ass., 151: 288-292, 1953.

2. Blumberg, H., Jänig, W. Changes of reflexes in vasoconstrictor neurons supplying the cat hindlimb following chronic nerve lesions: a model for studying mechanisms of reflex sympathetic dystrophy? J. Auton. Nerv. Syst., 7: 399-411, 1983.

3. Burchiel, K.J., Russell, L.C. Effects of potassium channel-blocking agents on spontaneous discharges from neuromas in rats. J. Neurosurg., 63: 246-249, 1985.

4. Cousins, M.J., Reeve, T.S., Glynn, C.J., Walsh, J.A., Cherry, D.A. Neurolytic lumbar sympathetic blockade: duration of denervation and relief of rest pain. Anaesth. Intens. Care, 7: 121, 1979.

5. Csillik, B., Knyihár-Csillik, E., Szucs, A. Treatment of chronic pain syndromes with iontophoresis of vinca alkaloids to the skin of patients. Neurosci. Letters, 31: 87-90, 1982.

6. DeSantis, M., Duckworth, J.W. Properties of primary afferent neurons from muscle which are spontaneously active after a lesion of their peripheral processes. Exp. Neurol., 75: 261-274, 1982.

7. Devor, M. Nerve pathophysiology and mechanisms of pain in causalgia. J. Auton. Nerv. Syst., 7: 371-384, 1983.

8. Devor, M., Govrin-Lippmann, R. Axoplasmatic transport block reduces ectopic impulse generation in injured peripheral nerves. Pain, 16: 73-85, 1983.

9. Devor, M., Govrin-Lippmann, R., Raber, P. Corticosteroids suppress ectopic neural discharge originating in experimental neuromas. Pain, 22: 127-137, 1985.

10. Devor, M., Jänig, W. Activation of myelinated afferents ending in a neuroma by stimulation of the sympathetic supply in the rat. Neurosci. Letters, 24: 43-47, 1981.

11. Devor, M., Wall, P.D. Reorganization of spinal cord sensory map after peripheral nerve injury. Nature, 276: 75-76, 1978.

12. Devor, M., Wall, P.D. Plasticity in the spinal cord sensory map following peripheral nerve injury in rats. J. Neurosci., 7: 679-684, 1981.

13. Ebert, M. H., Shader, R.I. Cardiovascular effects. In: Psychotropic Drug Side Effects: Clinical and Theoretical Perspectives (Shader, R.I., Di Mascio, A., eds.), Williams & Wilkins, Baltimore, pp. 149-163, 1970.

14. Fleckenstein, A., Burn, J.H. The effect of denervation on the action of sympathomimetic amines on the nictitating membrane. Br. J. Pharmacol., 8: 69-78, 1953.

15. Geffen, L. B., Livett, B.G., Rush, R.A. Immunohistochemical localization of protein components of catecholamine storage vesicles. J. Physiol. (Lond.), 204: 593-605, 1969.

16. Glynn, C.J., Basedow, R.W., Walsh, J.A. Pain relief following post-ganglionic blockade with IV guanethidine. Br. J. Anaesth., 53: 1297-1302, 1981.

17. Hannington-Kiff, J.G. Intravenous regional sympathetic block with guanethidine. Lancet, I: 1019-1020, 1974.

18. Hille, B. The selective inhibition of delayed potassium currents in nerve by tetraethylammonium ion. J. Gen. Physiol., 50: 1287-1302, 1967.

19. Hylden, J.L.K., Nahin, R.L., Dubner, R. Altered responses of nociceptive cat lamina I spinal dorsal horn neurons after chronic sciatic neuroma formation. Brain Res., 411: 341-350, 1987.

20. Innes, I. R., Kosterlitz, H.W. The effects of preganglionic and postganglionic denervation on the responses of the nictitating membrane to sympathomimetic substances. J. Physiol. (Lond.), 124: 25-43, 1954.

21. Jänig, W. Causalgia and reflex sympathetic dystrophy: in which way is the sympathetic nervous system involved? Trends Neurosci., 8: 471-477, 1985.

22. Janssen, P.A., Niemegers, C.J.E., Schellekens, H.L. Is it possible to predict the clinical effects of neuroleptic drugs (major tranquilizers) from animal data? Part I: "Neuroleptic activity spectra" for rats. Arzneim.-Forsch., 15: 104-117, 1965.

23. Jurna, I. Electrophysiological effects of antiepileptic drugs. In: Antiepileptic Drugs (Frey, H.-H. and J. Janz, eds.), Handbook of Experimental Pharmacology, Vol. 74, Springer, Berlin, pp. 611-658, 1985.

24. Kirk, E.J. Impulses in dorsal spinal nerve rootlets in cats and rabbits arising from dorsal root ganglia isolated from the periphery. J. Comp. Neurol., 2: 165-176, 1974.

25. Kleiman, A. Causalgia. Evidence of the existence of crossed sensory sympathetic fibers. Am. J. Surg., 87: 839-841, 1954.

26. Koppenhöfer, E. Die Wirkung von Tetraäthylammonium chlorid auf die Membranströme Ranvierscher Schnürringe von Xenopus laevis. Arch. Ges. Physiol., 293: 34-55, 1967.

27. Korenman, E.M.D., Devor, M. Ectopic adrenergic sensitivity in damaged peripheral nerve axons in the rat. Exp. Neurol., 72: 63-81, 1981.

28. Laduron, P., Belpaire, F. Transport of noradrenaline and dopamine-hydroxylase in sympathetic nerves. Life Sci., 7: 1-7, 1968.

29. Langer, S.Z., Trendelenburg, U. The onset of denervation sensitivity. J. Pharmacol. Exp. Ther., 151: 73-86, 1966.

30. Lisney, S.J.W. Changes in the somatotopic organization of the cat lumbar spinal cord following peripheral nerve transection and regeneration. Brain Res., 259: 31-39, 1983a.

31. Lisney, S.J.W. The cat lumbar spinal cord somatotopic map is unchanged after peripheral nerve crush and regeneration. Brain Res., 271: 166-169, 1983b.

32. Lockett, M.F. The effect of denervation on the response of the cat's nictitating membrane to sympathomimetic amines. Br. J. Pharmacol., 5: 485-496, 1950.

33. Loh, L., Nathan, P.W. Painful peripheral states and sympathetic blocks. J. Neurol. Neurosurg. Psychiat., 41: 664-671, 1978.

34. Peroutka, S.J., U'Prichard, D.C., Greenberg, D.A., Snyder, S.H. Neuroleptic drug interactions with norepinephrinealpha receptor binding sites in rat brain. Neuropharmacol., 16: 549-556, 1977.

35. Robson, R.D.M., Antonaccio, M.J., Fehn, P.A. Cardiovascular pharmacology of neuroleptics. In: Neuroleptics (Fielding, S. and H. Lal, eds.), Futura, New York, pp. 173-201, 1974.

36. Scadding, J.W. Development of ongoing activity, mechanosensitivity, and adrenaline sensitivity in severed peripheral nerve axons, Exp. Neurol., 73: 345-364, 1981.

37. Shumacker, H.B. Jr., Spiegal, I.J., Upjohn, R.H. Causalgia. I. The role of sympathetic interruption in the treatment. Surg. Gynec. Obstet., 86: 76-86, 1948.

38. Swerdlow, M. Anticonvulsant drugs used in the treatment of lancinating pain. Anaesthesia, 36: 1129-1132, 1981.

39. Swerdlow, M. Anticonvulsant drugs and chronic pain. Clin. Neuropharmacol., 7: 51-82, 1984.

40. Trendelenburg, U. Time course of changes in sensitivity after denervation of the nictitating membrane of the spinal cat. J. Pharmacol. Exp. Ther., 142: 335-342, 1963a.

41. Wall, P.D., Devor, M. The effect of peripheral nerve injury on dorsal root potentials and on transmission of afferent signals in the spinal cord. Brain Res., 209: 95-111, 1981.

42. Wall, P.D., Devor, M. Sensory afferent impulses from dorsal root ganglia as well as from the periphery in normal and nerve injured rats, Pain, 17: 321-339, 1983.

43. Wall, P.D., Devor, M., Inbal, R., Scadding, J.W., Schonfeld, D., Seltzer, Z., Tomkiewicz, M.M. Autotomy following peripheral nerve lesions: experimental anaesthesia dolorosa. Pain, 7: 103-113, 1979a.

44. Wall, P.D., Scadding, J.W., Tomkiewicz, M.M. The production and prevention of experimental anaesthesia dolorosa. Pain, 6: 175-182, 1979b.

45. Wall, P.D., Gutnick, M. Ongoing activity in peripheral nerves: the physiology and pharmacology of impulses originating from a neuroma. Exp. Neurol., 43: 580-593, 1974.

46. Walsh, J.A., Glynn, C.J., Cousins, M., Basedow, R.W. Blood flow, sympathetic activity and pain relief following lumbar sympathetic blockade or surgical sympathectomy. Anaesth. Intens. Care, 13: 18-24, 1984.

47. Weiner, N. Drugs that inhibit adrenergic nerves and block adrenergic receptors: In: Goodman and Gilman's The Pharmacological Basis of Therapeutics (Goodman Gilman, A., Goodman, L.S., Rall, T.W., Murad, F. eds.), Macmillan, New York, pp. 181-214, 1985.

48. Wiesenfeld-Hallin, Z., Hallin, R.G. Possible role of sympathetic activity in abnormal behavior of rats induced by lesion of the sciatic nerve. J. Auton. Nerv Syst., 7: 385-390, 1983.

49. Yaari, Y., Devor, M. Phenytoin suppresses spontaneous ectopic discharge in rat sciatic nerve neuromas. Neurosci. Letters, 58: 117-122, 1985.

9

CLINICAL AND NEUROPHYSIOLOGICAL OBSERVATIONS RELATING TO PATHOPHYSIOLOGICAL MECHANISMS IN REFLEX SYMPATHETIC DYSTROPHY

Erik Torebjörk

Acknowledgment: This work was supported by the Swedish Medical Research Council Project No. 14X-05206

INTRODUCTION

It is well known that sympathetic blocks may relieve pain in reflex sympathetic dystrophy (RSD), but the links between the sympathetic and nociceptive systems are poorly understood. One may speculate that there is a priori an increased sympathetic outflow, which is abolished by the block. Further, it is conceivable that various types of receptive nerve endings in the painful region may be abnormally reactive to sympathetic stimulation. It is also possible that the input from peripheral receptors, some of which may respond normally or abnormally to sympathetic stimulation, is abnormally treated in the central nervous system.

In attempts to test these possibilities six patients with reflex sympathetic dystrophy have been studied. Following previous injury, all had spontaneous burning pain and pronounced allodynia, particularly to tactile stimuli and cold. The painful regions in their hands or feet did not follow the boundaries of any particular nerve or segment. Sympathetic blocks temporarily relieved the pain in all patients.

METHODS

Measurements of Sensory Thresholds

The sensory thresholds for warmth, cold, heat pain and cold pain were tested using the Marstock method (4). Tactile thresholds and thresholds for pain induced by mechanical stimuli were determined using a plastic probe of 2 mm diameter mounted on a Bruel and Kjaer vibrator, driven by half-cycle pulses (10).

Microneurography and Intraneural Microstimulation

Nerve fibre action potentials were recorded with tungsten microelectrodes inserted percutaneously into cutaneous fascicles of the medial, radial or peroneal nerve, supplying symptomatic skin. Details of the microelectrodes and the recording and display system have been given elsewhere (8). The same electrodes were also used to deliver electric shocks into the nerve, a technique termed intraneural microstimulation (24).

Topical Application of Noradrenaline

Noradrenaline (NA) was applied to the skin either by iontophoresis of NA 0.2 mg/ml in an area of 2 cm^2 with a DC-current of 1-2 mA for 2 minutes, or by intracutaneous injection of NA 1-5 ug.

Compression Nerve Block

In one patient who had symptoms on the dorsum of the hand, the superficial branch of the radial nerve supplying this area was partially blocked by prolonged pressure for up to 50 min. A 2 cm wide band was placed across the wrist proximal to symptomatic skin and loaded by 4-6 kg. Sensory thresholds for touch, temperature and pain were tested throughout the course of the block.

RESULTS

Recording of Sympathetic Outflow

Microneurographic recordings of multifibre sympathetic outflow to symptomatic skin areas were performed at room temperature in four patients.

The sympathetic discharges were organized in irregular bursts of impulses, which were greatly influenced by the attentative state of the subject. Thus, the number of sympathetic nerve impulses per burst and the number of bursts were increased by arousal stimuli and mental stress. This is typical also in normal subjects (6,7,9), and no gross increase in the overall sympathetic activity to symptomatic skin was observed in these patients, as compared to what is usually seen in normal subjects. Furthermore, no obvious changes in the amount or pattern of skin sympathetic activity were observed in one patient after he had been temporarily relieved from spontaneous pain by transcutaneous electrical nerve stimulation, as compared with pre-stimulation control with spontaneous pain. Thus, the results from these few experiments failed to support the notion that the sympathetic outflow would be greatly enhanced in patients with RSD. However, it should be pointed out that no attempts were made to differentiate between sudomotor versus vasomotor outflow, and no systematic experiments were performed to test whether reflex activity in these subsystems were normal or not. Thus, the apparently normal spontaneous pattern of the overall sympathetic outflow to the skin in these patients does by no means exclude dysfunction of either sudomotor or vasomotor reflexes.

**Allodynia Following Typical Applications
of Noradrenaline**

In four patients who were partially relieved from allodynia and spontaneous pain by sympathetic blocks or sympathectomy, topical application of noradrenaline was performed either by iontophoresis or by intracutaneous injection. In all patients, application of noradrenaline in previously symptomatic skin regions results in revival of allodynia to tactile stimuli and even spontaneous burning pain. In two subjects tested, there was also allodynia to cold and heat stimuli. The allodynia appeared with a latency of 3 to 30 min. after application of noradrenaline, and lasted for 1.5 to 2.5 hours. The area of allodynia spread beyond the application zone for noradrenaline, and at its peak, it could cover an area 10 to 20 times larger than the infiltration zone.

Such reactions to noradrenaline were not observed in a control of 15 normal subjects, none of whom developed allodynia or spontaneous pain following noradrenaline injections.

Nerve Fibre Blocks

It has been shown in direct microneurographic recordings from the superficial nerve in normal human subjects that firm compression of the nerve at wrist level will cause a progressive block of impulse conduction first in large and then in thin myelinated nerve fibres (22). This is accompanied by loss of tactile sensibility, soon followed by loss of sensation of cold (7,13). At this stage, when all myelinated fibres are blocked, unmyelinated (C) fibres are still conducting, and sensations of warmth and delayed burning pain are preserved. This kind of nerve compression block was used to study which fibre types were involved in the production of noradrenaline-induced allodynia. A patient who was partially relieved from causalgia in her left hand by sympathectomy served as experimental subject. Noradrenaline was injected intracutaneously within the innervation territory of the radial nerve on the dorsum of her left hand. When allodynia to tactile and cold stimuli started to develop, firm compression was applied on the radial nerve at wrist level. As the tactile sensibility disappeared during the block, so did allodynia to touch, and when cold sensibility disappeared, allodynia to cold was greatly reduced. After release of nerve compression, allodynia to tactile and cold stimuli reappeared in parallel with recovery of tactile and cold sensibility. Experiments of this kind, which were repeated ten times in this patient with similar results, indicate that myelinated fibres are involved in the production of allodynia to touch and cold, and that fairly large myelinated fibres account for the allodynia to touch. Interestingly, this patient also had allodynia to moderately warm stimuli. Her heat pain threshold was as low as 33°C and dropped further down to 31°C after noradrenaline injection. Such allodynia to warmth persisted at a time when sensations of touch and cold were completely abolished by nerve compression, indicating that allodynia to warmth was mediated by C fibres (23).

Intraneural Microstimulation

Intraneural electrical microstimulation in cutaneous fascicles of the median nerve at 5 Hz in four normal human subjects evoked tactile sensations at liminal intensity for conscious detection in about 80% of 290 tests, and pain as the threshold sensation in only 20% of the tests (20). In two patients with RSD and allodynia to touch, intraneural stimulation at 5 Hz in cutaneous fascicles of the median nerve supplying symptomatic skin evoked pain as the first threshold sensation in 90% of 30 tests. Furthermore, the magnitude of pain increased with increase in stimulus frequency, and became almost intolerable at 50 to 100 Hz. Sustained high frequency stimulation for many seconds evoked sustained severe pain, without the rapid decay observed in normal subjects (26).

Post-ischemic Paresthesiae

It is common experience that release of an arm cuff inflated above systolic pressure for 15-20 min. at the level of the upper arm will result in post-ischemic paresthesiae projected mainly to the hand. Such paresthesiae have been described as tingling, buzzing or pricking (14), and albeit intense, they are well tolerated by normal subjects. In two patients with RSD and allodynia to touch in the hand, post-ischemic paresthesia projected to the hand after relapse of a cuff inflated in upper arm for 15 minutes was excruciatingly painful.

DISCUSSION

Even though the presented data are obtained from a limited number of patients, the observations yield some interesting insights into pathophysiological mechanisms involved in RSD. One striking finding was that topical application of noradrenaline to symptomatic skin in patients with RSD produced allodynia and spontaneous pain, whereas no such effects were observed in normal subjects. A possible explanation is that sufficient concentrations of noradrenaline would increase the excitability of certain types of nerve endings in the periphery, thereby increasing the afferent barrage elicited by various types of skin stimuli. Indeed, reports from experiments both in normal humans (28) and in cats (17,19) indicate that various types of low threshold mechanoreceptors in the skin are activated by sympathetic stimulation. It is conceivable that such responsiveness to sympathetic outflow is enhanced in patients with RSD. However, direct data from microneurographic recordings in patients to support this hypothesis are still lacking.

The other striking finding was that allodynia to tactile stimuli and cold was mediated by myelinated fibres, as indicated by the results from the nerve compression blocks. This notion was further supported by the observation that intraneural microstimulation at threshold intensity for detection evoked pain rather than tactile sensations in RSD patients. Since large diameter fibres have lower electrical thresholds than thin fibres, many of these pain sensations from threshold stimulation must have been evoked by activation of large myelinated fibres. In line with this reasoning is the finding that 50 to 100 Hz intraneural stimulation elicited severe, sustained pain. It is known from direct recordings in humans that unmyelinated (C) fibres cannot follow such high frequencies for more than a few seconds, and that C fibre mediated pain from such stimulation rapidly fades away (25). Finally, it was observed that post-ischemic paresthesiae were severely painful in RSD patients, in contrast to what is normally perceived. Microneurographic records in normal human nerves have shown that post-ischemic paresthesiae are mediated from ectopic impulse generation in myelinated but not in unmyelinated nerve fibres (15). If this is so in patients with RSD it would again implicate myelinated fibers in the production of severe pain.

Taken together, all these findings indicate that myelinated fibres, many of which normally mediate tactile sensations (7,13,16,24), instead elicit pain in RSD patients. This notion receives support from several other clinical observations (2,11,12,27), and implies abnormal function within the central nervous system, probably at the level of the spinal cord (29). Thus, an input from low threshold mechanoreceptors with myelinated fibres, some of which may be sensitive to noradrenaline, is assumed to cause intense pain because of disinhibition or facilitation within the central nervous system. This hypothesis does not necessarily require that the sympathetic outflow to symptomatic skin is increased, and the few nerve recordings performed so far in patients with RSD have failed to show any obvious sympathetic hyperactivity. Furthermore, the presumed hypersensitivity to noradrenaline may not be restricted to nerve endings with myelinated fibres. As illustrated in this report, one RSD patient had severe allodynia to mild warming. Her heat pain threshold was as low as 34°C and was further lowered to 31°C by noradrenaline injections. Since her heat pain threshold remained abnormally low during nerve compression block of impulse conduction in myelinated fibres, her allodynia to warmth was mediated by unmyelinated C fibres. If C polymodal nociceptors mediate heat pain in this patient, as in normal subjects (7), her C nociceptors were greatly sensitized, since C nociceptors in normal human subjects have thresholds above 41°C (26). That chronic sensitization of C polymodal nociceptors can occur in humans under pathological conditions has only recently been shown (3). Thus, even though little or no sensitizing effect of sympathetic stimulation has been observed on the excitability of the nociceptors in animal experiments (1,18,21), it is conceivable that such phenomena contribute to pain and allodynia in patients with severe causalgia.

REFERENCES

1. Barasi, S., Lynn, B. Effects of sympathetic stimulation on mechanoreceptive and nociceptive afferent units from the rabbit pinna. Brain Res., 378: 21-27, 1986.

2. Campbell, J.N., Raja, S.N., Meyer, R.A. Mackinnon, S.E. Myelinated afferents signal the hyperalgesia associated with nerve injury. Pain, 32: 89-94 1988.

3.   Cline, M.A., Ochoa, J.L., Torebjörk, H.E.   Chronic hyperalgesia and skin warming caused by sensitized C nociceptors. Brain, in press, 1989.

4.   Fruhstorfer, H., Lindblom, U., Schmidt, W.G.   Method for quantitative estimation of thermal thresholds in patients. J. Neurol. Neurosurg. Psychiatr., 39: 1071-1075, 1976.

5.   Hallin, R.G., Torebjork, H.E.   Studies on cutaneous A and C fibre afferents, skin nerve blocks and perception. In: Y. Zotterman (Ed.) Sensory Functions of the Skin in Primates, Oxford Univ. Press, Oxford, pp. 137-149, 1979.

6.   Hallin, R.G., Torebjörk, H.E.   Afferent and efferent C units recorded from human skin nerves in situ. Acta Soc. Med. Upsal., 75: 277-281, 1970.

7.   Hallin, R.G., Torebjork, H.E.   Single unit sympathetic activity in human skin nerves during rest and various manoeuvres. Acta Physiol. Scand., 92: 303-317, 1976.

8.   Hagbarth, K.-E., Hongell, A., Hallin, R.G., Torebjörk, H.E.   Afferent impulses in median nerve fascicles evoked by tactile stimuli of the human hand. Brain Res., 24: 423-442, 1970.

9.   Hagbarth, K.E., Hallin, R.G., Hongell, A., Torebjörk, H.E., Wallin, B.G.   General characteristics of sympathetic activity in human skin nerves. Acta Physiol. Scand., 84: 164-176, 1972.

10.   Lindblom, U.   Touch perception threshold in human glabrous skin in terms of displacement amplitude on stimulation with single mechanical pulses. Brain Res., 82: 205-210, 1974.

11.   Lindblom, U., Verillo, V.T.   Sensory functions in chronic neuralgia. J. Neurol. Neurosurg. Psychiat., 42: 422-435, 1979.

12.   Loh, L., Nathan, P.W.   Painful peripheral states and sympathetic blocks. J. Neurol. Neurosurg. Psychiat., 41: 664-671, 1978.

13.   Mackenzie, R.A., Burke, D., Skuse, N.F., Lehlean, A.K.   Fibre function and perception during cutaneous nerve block. J. Neurol. Neurosurg.

Psychiat., 38: 865-873, 1975.

14. Merrington, W.R., Nathan, P.W. A study of post-ischaemic paraesthesiae. J. Neurol. Neurosurg. Psychiat., 12: 1-18, 1949.

15. Ochoa, J.L., Torebjörk, H.E. Paraesthesiae from ectopic impulse generation in human sensory nerves. Brain, 103: 835-853, 1980.

16. Ochoa, J.L., Torebjörk, H.E. Sensations evoked by intraneural microstimulation of single mechanoreceptor units innervating the human hand. J. Physiol. (Lond.), 342: 633-654, 1983.

17. Pierce, J.P., Roberts, W.J. Sympathetically induced changes in the responses of guard hair and type II receptors in the cat. J. Physiol. (Lond.), 314: 411-428, 1981.

18. Roberts, W.J., Elardo, S.M. Sympathetic activation of A-delta nociceptors. Somatosens. Res., 3: 33-44, 1985.

19. Roberts, W.J., Elardo, S.M., King, K.A. Sympathetically-induced changes in the responses of slowly-adapting type I receptors in cat skin. Somatosens. Res., 2: 223-236, 1985.

20. Schady, W.J.L., Torebjork, H.E., Ochoa, J.L. Peripheral projections of nerve fibres in the human median nerve. Brain Res., 277: 249-261, 1983.

21. Shea, V.K., Perl, E.R. Failure of sympathetic stimulation to effect responsiveness of rabbit polymodal nociceptors. J. Neurophysiol., 54: 513-520, 1985.

22. Torebjörk, H.E., Hallin, R.G. Perceptual changes accompanying controlled preferential blocking of A and C fibre responses in intact human skin nerves. Exp. Brain Res., 16: 321-332, 1973.

23. Torebjörk, H.E., Hallin, R.G. Microneurographic studies of peripheral pain mechanisms in man. In: J.J. Bonica et al., (Eds.) Advances in

Pain Research and Therapy, Vol. 3, Raven Press, New York, pp. 121-131, 1979.

24.　Torebjörk, H.E., Ochoa, J. Specific sensations evoked by activity in single identified sensory units in man. Acta Physiol. Scand., 110: 445-447, 1980.

25.　Torebjörk, H.E., Schady, W., Ochoa, J.L. A new method for demonstration of central effects of analgesic agents in man. J. Neurol. Neurosurg. Psychiat., 47: 862-869, 1984a.

26.　Torebjörk, H.E., LaMotte, R.H., Robinson, C.J. Peripheral neural correlates of magnitude of cutaneous pain and hyperalgesia: Simultaneous recordings in humans of sensory judgments of pain and evoked responses in nociceptors with C-fibers. J. Neurophysiol., 51: 325-339, 1984b.

27.　Wallin, B.G., Torebjörk, H.E., Hallin, R.G. Preliminary observations on the pathophysiology of hyperalgesia in the causalgic pain syndrome. In Y. Zotterman (Ed.) Sensory Functions of the Skin in Primates. Pergamon Press, Oxford, pp. 489-499, 1976.

28.　Wiesenfeld-Hallin, Z., Hallin, R.G. The influence of the sympathetic system on mechanoreception and nociception. A review. Hum. Neurobiol., 3: 41-46, 1984.

29.　Woolf, C.J. Evidence for a central component in post-injury pain hypersensitivity. Nature (Lond.), 306: 686-688, 1983.

10

MECHANISMS AND ROLE OF PERIPHERAL BLOOD FLOW DYSREGULATION IN PAIN SENSATION AND EDEMA IN REFLEX SYMPATHETIC DYSTROPHY

H. Blumberg, H.J. Griesser, M.E. Hornyak

The term "reflex sympathetic dystrophy" (RSD) is used to denote a number of various diseases affecting the extremities such as Sudeck's atrophy, causalgia, shoulder-hand syndrome, and algodystrophy (11,16,18,25,41). As evidenced in these presentations, there have so far been no generally accepted theories explaining the basic pathophysiological mechanisms of RSD.

In this paper we introduce ideas concerning the pathophysiology of RSD, particularly as regards the development of spontaneous pain and edema. These ideas are based on the clinical picture of RSD and on human and animal experimental findings related to the sympathetic control of skin blood flow in RSD-patients (3,5,7,9).

Clinical Symptoms - The Triad of RSD

The clinical symptoms of RSD vary. The major symptoms are pain in and swelling of a distal extremity. According to the literature (9,33,50) and unpublished results of our clinical investigations in 144 RSD patients (78 female, 66 male, mean age 51 years), the symptoms, which may all occur at the first day of onset of RSD, can be divided into three groups:

I. <u>Autonomic</u>. The skin of the affected distal extremity is noticeably warmer in most cases, but is sometimes colder than the unaffected extremity. Usually, edema is generalized in the distal extremity and is most prominent on the dorsal surface. It is often combined with reddened or cyanotic skin and with hypohydrosis or hyperhydrosis (sympathetic changes).

II. Motor. Active movements, especially complex movements (making a fist, positioning first and fifth fingers opposite one another) are disturbed. Muscle strength is often diminished in all motor functions of the distal extremity (paresis). Passive movement disorders, if not a direct consequence of trauma or surgery, may appear after weeks or months. Tremor in the affected extremity is not uncommon.

III. Sensory. Regardless of the cause of the RSD, most cases show signs of hypo or hyperesthesia, hypo or hyperalgesia, and less frequently, allodynia (pain resulting from slight, brief touch or from cold). These, along with a spontaneous pain syndrome (see below), make up the group of sensory disturbances. Skin sensory disturbances, with the exception of allodynia, chiefly affect the palm of the hand.

Thus, in the very early stage of RSD there is a triad of autonomic, motor, and sensory disturbances. In most cases, all components of the triad affect the entire distal extremity. The generalized occurrence of such a triad can be regarded as the main diagnostic criterion for RSD (9). In addition to these clinical findings, a comparative measurement of *all finger or toe tip temperatures*, can provide objective data on the disturbed skin circulation, supporting the diagnosis. In 75% of 113 RSD-patients in whom the upper extremity was affected, we found that there was a *systematic side difference* in skin temperature (all points on the affected side exhibited either higher (n = 62) or lower (n = 23) temperatures when compared with corresponding sites on the healthy side; unpublished results).

Various factors can provoke RSD as presented in Chapter 2: minor trauma (9,11,25,28,32), partial nerve lesion or bone fracture (18,24,30,35,37,42,44,49,50), atraumatic nerve lesion such as herpes zoster (15,36,43,48), or a visceral lesion such as myocardial infarction (1,10,14,43,51). Regardless of the cause or location of the precipitating event, the symptoms of RSD almost always appear in the distal part of an extremity. Elevating the affected extremity diminishes both the swelling and the pain. Sympatholytic therapy applied soon after onset of the disease, helps the pain syndrome with subsequent improvement in other symptoms (1,2,9,17,21,22,25,27,28,29,34,38,50).

Pain Syndrome in RSD

Pain associated with RSD is experienced even under resting conditions (spontaneous pain), during physical strain and under orthostatic conditions (strain-dependent pain), or during movement of joints (movement related pain). Spontaneous pain is typically more severe during the night. Elevating the extremity often alleviates spontaneous pain. In most cases, spontaneous pain in the distal extremity is experienced diffusely and deeply. Less frequently it occurs diffusely and superficially with palmar or plantar predominance. Neither pain is confined to innervation zones of single nerves or dermatomes. The spontaneous and strain dependent pain is described as throbbing, aching, shooting, stabbing, or (even in cases without concomitant nerve lesion) burning.

The history of RSD patients in most cases reveals a noxious, painful event preceding the onset of RSD. Typically, the pain experienced in RSD is different from the original pain sensation and is in a different location. The latter point should be considered an indication that RSD has developed (i.e., local pressure pain under a cast applied for a fractured radius, which later turns into deep diffuse pain in the entire hand). A similar presentation with full RSD, followed within hours of a single painful injection in the arm (9).

Mechanisms of Pain in RSD

A number of theories have been proposed regarding the mechanism of pain in RSD. Most of them attribute the pain to pathophysiological changes following a nerve lesion. Examples are: spontaneous activity of lesioned nociceptive axons (3,6,8); ephaptic transmission between lesioned nerve fibres (3,4); or foci of abnormal activity of dorsal horn neurons of the pain system (47). For two reasons, however, they are not likely to be the source of pain in most cases of RSD. First, RSD pain is felt diffusely (deeply or superficially) in the distal extremity, unrelated to the innervation zone of the lesioned nerve (11,35,38,50). Secondly, RSD pain associated with nerve lesions is of the same quality and has the same spatial distribution as pain in cases without nerve lesion; for example following a minor trauma (9) or a visceral lesion (1,10,14,43,51).

Sudeck (45,46) assumed that collateral inflammation following trauma, especially a bone fracture, was responsible for the symptoms of RSD. However, such mechanisms cannot be considered if there has been no trauma and if the affected limb is colder at the outset (9).

Another theory was recently proposed by Roberts (39). Based upon experimental findings in animals, he considered *sensitized spinal cord wide dynamic range neurons* (WDR-neurons) to be the source of spontaneous pain and allodynia. Mechanoreceptive and nociceptive inputs converge onto these neurons. The spinal neurons may become sensitized following a noxious event. This sensitization is maintained by a mechanoreceptive input, which in turn is produced by the spontaneous activity of sympathetic fibres, which excite mechano-afferent structures in the skin. This finally leads to spontaneous pain and allodynia, initially located at the site of the original noxious event. Pain and allodynia may spread, as neighboring neurons at the spinal cord level also become sensitized. Sympatholytic therapy can interrupt sympathetic excitation of mechanoreceptors, which reduces the afferent input and reverses the sensitization of the WDR-neurons. Such mechanisms may play a role in RSD with spontaneous pain and allodynia. They are not likely to exist, however, if there is no allodynia. Neither is this likely if there is a lesion at a proximal site of the extremity, with spontaneous pain as well as the other symptoms of RSD confined to the distal region of the affected extremity (9).

There is no theory that explains the mechanisms underlying the generalized swelling of distal extremities in cases of RSD with different etiologies. This major symptom of RSD may occur at the first day of onset of the disease in the absence of a nerve lesion or a local trauma at the distal extremity and without previous immobilisation (9).

None of the foregoing notions satisfactorily explain why elevation of the affected extremity can reduce pain and swelling in RSD (9,11,32,35,50). This point brings into consideration the dysregulation of blood flow as a causative factor in the etiology of pain and edema in RSD.

Such a hypothesis ideally should provide answers to the following questions:

1.) What are the mechanisms that initiate RSD?

2.) Why is it that similar events, even in the same patient, do not always bring on RSD?

3.) Why is pain and generalized swelling located in the distal extremities, regardless of the precipitating factor or its location?

4.) What are the possible mechanisms responsible for "spontaneous" activation of nociceptors in these regions?

5.) Why is it that sympatholytic therapy is able to cure the entire syndrome?

6.) How does elevating the affected extremity reduce pain and swelling?

Hypothesis on the Pathophysiological Mechanisms of Pain and Edema in RSD

This hypothesis extends the ideas formulated by Livingston (28), who assumes a vicious circle taking place in RSD. Figure 1 gives a schematic representation of these concepts.

HYPOTHESIS ABOUT DEVELOPMENT OF RSD - PAIN SYNDROME

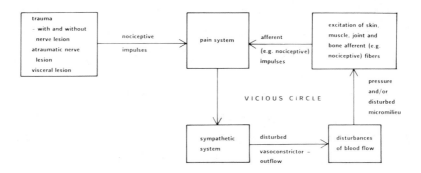

Fig. 1.   Diagram of hypothesis regarding the development of pain syndrome in RSD

A common factor among the various causes of RSD (for example, trauma with an without nerve lesion, visceral lesion) is the occurrence of a noxious event, which induces nociceptive impulses. These reach the central nervous structures of the pain system and thereby reflexly influence (e.g., at the spinal cord) the discharge pattern of sympathetic preganglionic neurons. If the integrative function of preganglionic vasoconstrictor neurons happens to be in vulnerable condition, the nociceptive impulses may finally produce a disturbed vasoconstrictor outflow. This disrupts blood flow regulation at the peripheral microcirculatory level. If the activity of vasoconstrictor neurons supplying the veins becomes higher than that of those supplying the arteries, the venous return is diminished. As a result, the capillary filtration pressure increases, edema forms, and the micromileiu becomes disturbed. This may lead to the excitation of afferent fibres (e.g., nociceptors) of affected tissues (e.g., skin, bones), which in turn reflexively maintains the disturbed vasoconstrictor outflow. If peripherally nociceptors are excited, this produces neurogenic inflammation, further supporting edema. A vicious circle has started.

The core of the hypothesis is the assumption that pain sensation in RSD is the result of peripheral nociceptor activity secondary to dysregulation of peripheral blood flow. These changes are induced by a dysfunction of sympathetic vasoconstrictor neurons supplying the skin vessels, resulting in superficial pain, and deep tissue vessels (e.g., bone vessels) causing deep pain.

The following are posited answers to the questions stated above.

1.) If different factors can cause RSD, it seems justified to assume that they have something in common which can start the syndrome. A noxious event is one such common factor in most cases of RSD. Due to this event, impulses are generated in primary afferent nociceptors, which project to the dorsal horn of spinal cord. This activity reflexly influences the discharge pattern of sympathetic preganglionic vasoconstrictor neurons.

2.) If at a synaptic level the integrative function of these preganglionic neurons happens to be in a so-called "vulnerable condition," the occurring nociceptor input may alter the ability of descending systems to control the discharge pattern of these neurons. This finally results in a disturbed vasoconstrictor outflow, which influences the peripheral blood flow at the microcirculatory level.

3.) A cause for dysregulation of peripheral blood flow is an imbalance between the pattern or activity (tone) of vasoconstrictor neurons supplying arteries (AVT) and those supplying veins (VVT). When the VVT is higher than the AVT, venous return is impaired in the affected regions, capillary filtration pressure increases, and edema results. This leads to higher interstitial pressure, which may excite peripheral nociceptors. Alternatively or additionally, increased filtration from blood vessels may induce disturbances of the micromilieu which "chemically" excite nociceptors. Independent of the actual mechanism causing nociceptor activation, this activation supports edema formation, since a "neurogenic inflammation" is induced (13). Excitation of nociceptors then reflexly maintains the disturbance of vasoconstrictor outflow. A vicious circle has begun.

The regions affected most are those in which there is a high density of capillaries and vasoconstrictor innervation; for example, the distal parts of the extremities (hand and foot). The dorsal areas of these regions will reveal most of the edema, since there the skin is not tightly attached to the underlying tissue.

In contrast, afferent receptors in palmar sites will be most affected by the increased interstitial pressure, since there, the skin is tightly attached to the underlying tissue. This may cause sensory dysfunction of various kinds (e.g., hypoesthesia and hyperalgesia) and activation of nociceptors or even larger myelinated afferents (WDR neuron afferents). Therefore, if the vasoconstrictor outflow to the skin is disturbed in this way, superficial pain will be primarily sensed in the palm of the hand. If the vasoconstrictor outflow to the deep tissues (e.g., bones) is disturbed in the same manner, diffuse and deep pain will occur. Deep tissue edema will have the greatest sensory consequences in the distal parts of an extremity, since there, especially in small bones, a small volume of filtrate will result in the greatest increase in interstitial pressure.

During erect posture, hydrostatic pressure is highest in the distal parts of an extremity, constraining venous return. Consequently, pain and edema are also more distal.

Pain sensation and edema are not confined to zones of single nerves or dermatomes but are generalized, since the sympathetic supply affects the blood flow in these regions in a generalized way.

4.) Sympatholytic therapy interrupts the abnormal venoconstrictor outflow, which improves venous return and so lowers interstitial pressure. Nociceptor excitation is thereby reduced. This interrupts the vicious circle.

In general, therefore, any treatment which improves the microcirculation to enhance venous return, will reduce pain sensation and edema.

Discussion

The idea that nociceptor impulses can cause RSD is consistent with clinical observations and a recognition that most RSD cases are preceded by a noxious event.

Crucial for the development of the disease is a disturbed sympathetic outflow which is initiated by these nociceptor impulses. The cause for increased neural activity of the sympathetic vasoconstrictor system appears to be a central spinal "vulnerability" at the time of the noxious event, as described by Roberts in Chapter 7. This sheds some light on the question as to why the same type of lesion initiates RSD in some but not most individuals. Thus, psychological, medical, constitutional, or other factors, do not seem to be primarily involved, but their influence on spinal sensitisation processes cannot be ruled out.

There are no experimental data to confirm the theory regarding the relationship between nociceptor input and onset of RSD. The same applies for the assumption of an imbalance between AVT and VVT. Though the literature does not make a differentiation between various subsets of vasoconstrictor neurons, there is no doubt that both arteries and veins are innervated by vasoconstrictor neurons (12,20,23,40,52). Since differential resistance (arteries) or capacitance changes (veins), are controlled via the sympathetic vasoconstrictor neurons (20,31), it is reasonable to assume that the activity of the two types of neurons is controlled separately at the central nervous level.

Ficat and Arlet (19) found in 29 RSD patients that there was increased bone pressure with diminished venous return from bone circulation. They interpreted their findings to be the result of disturbed sympathetic control of bone vessels. We regard this increase in bone pressure as the most likely mechanism for spontaneous deep pain in early stages of RSD. Indirect evidence supports this idea, since hyperemia and edema in bones is a common finding in RSD (16).

Skin vasoconstrictor neurons of nerve lesioned cats undergo a qualitative change in their reflex pattern upon baroreceptor, chemoreceptor, and on nociceptor stimulation (3,5,7). This change occurred in lesioned as well as intact skin nerves of the affected extremity, indicating that peripheral events can alter the reflex control of the vasoconstrictor neurons at the central nervous level (e.g., spinal cord).

Experimental investigations of RSD in the upper extremity showed, in accordance with others (15,26,33,50), that the reflex control of arterial skin blood flow in response to thermal load is disturbed on the affected side (9). In response to whole body cooling, hands excluded, blood flow decreased either faster or more slowly on the affected side than on the healthy side. In most cases the entire distal extremity showed the same abnormal blood flow reaction. This generalized abnormal reaction occurred independent of the site or causative factor of RSD. It was concluded that these findings are based upon an abnormal state of reflex excitability of skin vasoconstrictor neurons.

Up to now it has not been fully understood how a sympathetic block could help in cases of RSD, especially in those with warmed skin (low vasoconstrictor activity). Considering, however, that a functional imbalance between arteriolar and venoconstrictor activity (for example, VVT being higher than AVT) is causing the superficial and/or deep edema, it becomes clear why this therapy can be successful. In cases with an extremity that is either too cool, too warm, or without signs of disturbed arterial skin blood flow, and painful (either superficial or deep pain), this therapy interrupts the abnormal venoconstrictor activity of skin and/or deep tissue (e.g., bone) veins. Venous return increases and the interstitial pressure and consequently "spontaneous" activity of the afferent fibres (e.g., nociceptors) is thus reduced. This gives relief of pain. When the vicious circle is interrupted, the pain as well as the edema disappear and the syndrome may be cured.

Another finding consistent with this hypothesis is the improvement in symptoms of RSD that occur when the limb is elevated (reducing the hydrostatic pressure). If, however, VVT is much higher than AVT, elevation may not be able to alleviate the pain. On the other hand, increasing either the blood flow (e.g., physical strain) or the hydrostatic pressure (orthostatic conditions) will enhance the symptoms. In cases where VVT is only slightly higher than AVT, symptoms will be mild and will only be enhanced by these mechanisms. Such mild cases are likely to escape the correct diagnosis of RSD unless it is recognized that the triad (i.e., autonomic, motor and sensory disturbances) occurs in a generalized way in the distal extremity. Additional evidence to support a diagnosis of RSD can be obtained with a comparative measurement of all finger or toe tips temperature of both sides. This measurement is especially helpful in cases with mild symptoms if a systematic side difference of skin temperature is found. In general, this finding can be taken as an indication that the sympathetic vasoconstrictor system is disturbed.

REFERENCES

1. Askey, J.M. The syndrome of painful disability of the shoulder and hand complicating coronary occlusion. Am Heart J, 22: 1-12, 1941.

2. Bentley, J.B., Hameroff, S.R. Diffuse reflex sympathetic dystrophy, Anesthesiology, 53: 256-257, 1980.

3. Blumberg, H., Jänig, W. Neurophysiological analysis of afferent and efferent (sympathetic) fibers in skin nerves with experimentally produced neuromata. In: J. Siegfried, M. Zimmermann, (Eds.), Phantom and Stump Pain, Springer-Verlag, Berlin, Heidelberg, New York, pp. 15-31, 1981.

4. Blumberg, H., Jänig, W. Activation of fibres via experimentally produced stump neuromata of skin nerves: ephaptic transmission or retrograde sprouting? Exp Neurol, 76: 468-482, 1982.

5. Blumberg, H., Jänig, W. Changes of reflexes in vasoconstrictor neurons supplying the cat hindlimb following chronic nerve lesions: a model for studying mechanisms of reflex sympathetic dystrophy? J Auton Nerv Syst, 7: 399-411, 1983.

6. Blumberg, H., Jänig, W. Discharge pattern of afferent fibers from a neuroma. Pain, 20: 335-353, 1984.

7. Blumberg, H., Jänig, W. Reflex patterns in postganglionic vasoconstrictor neurons following chronic nerve lesions. J Aut Nerv Syst, 14: 157-180, 1985.

8. Blumberg, H., Jänig, W. Changes in primary afferent axons following lesions of their axons. In: L.M. Pubols (Ed.), Effects of injury on spinal and trigeminal somatosensory systems. Alan R. Riss, New York, pp. 85-92, 1987.

9. Blumberg, H. Zur Entstehung und Therapie des Schmerzsyndroms bei der sympathischen Reflex-dystrophy. Der Schmerz, 2: 125-143, 1988.

10. Boas, E.P., Levy, H. Extracardiac determinations of the site and radiation of pain in angina with special reference to shoulder pain. Am Heart J, 14: 540-554, 1937.

11. Bonica, J.J. Causalgia and other reflex sympathetic dystrophies. In: J.J. Bonica (Ed.), Advances in Pain Research and Therapy, Vol. 3, Raven Press, New York, pp. 141-166, 1979.

12. Browse, N.L., Lorentz, R.R., Shepherd, J.T. Response of capacity and resistance vessels of dog's limb to sympathetic nerve stimulation. Amer J Physiol, 210: 95-102, 1966.

13. Chahl, L.A., Szolcsányi, J., Lembeck, F. (Eds.) Antidromic vasodilatation and neurogenic inflammation, Akadémiai Kiadó, Budapest, 1984.

14. Chitwood, W.R. The Importance of recognizing post-infarctional shoulder-hand syndrome. N Engl J Med, 243: 813-814, 1951.

15. De Takats, G., Miller, D.S. Post-traumatic dystrophy of the extremities. Arch Surg, 46: 469-479, 1943.

16. Doury, P., Dirheimer, Y., Pattin, S. Algodystrophy. Springer, Berlin, 1981.

17. Dunningham, T.H. The treatment of Sudeck's atrophy in the upper limb by sympathetic blockade. Injury, 12: 139-144, 1980.

18. Evans J.A. Reflex sympathetic dystrophy. Surg Clin North Amer, 26: 780-790, 1946.

19. Ficat, R.P., Arlet, J. Ischemia and necroses of bone (translated from the French by D. S. Hungerford). Williams & Wilkins, Baltimore, 1980.

20. Hainsworth, R. Vascular capacitance: Its control and importance. Rev Physiol Biochem Pharmacol, 105: 101-173, 1986.

21. Hannington-Kiff, J.G. Relief of Sudeck's atrophy by regional intravenous Guanethidine. Lancet I, 28: 1132-1133, 1977.

22. Hathaway, B.N., Hill, G.E., Ohmura, A. Centrally induced sympathetic dystrophy of the upper extremity. Anesth Analg, 57: 373-374, 1978.

23. Hottenstein, O.D., Kreulen, D.L. Comparison of the frequency dependence of venous and arterial responses to sympathetic nerve stimulation in guinea-pigs. J Physiol, 384: 153-167, 1987.

24. Kleinert, H.E., Cole, N.M., Wayne, L., Harvey, R., Kutz, J.E., Atasoy, E. Post-traumatic sympathetic dystrophy. Orthop Clin North Am, 4: 917-928, 1973.

25. Lankford, L.L. Reflex sympathetic dystrophy. In: G.E. Omer, M. Spinner, (Eds.), Management of peripheral nerve problems. Saunders, Philadelphia, pp. 216-244, 1980.

26. Leriche, R. Sur les déséquilibres vaso-moteurs post-traumatiques primitifs des extrémités. Lyon Cirurgical, 20: 746-753, 1923.

27. Leriche, R. Chirurgie des Schmerzes (aus dem Französischen übersetzt von E. Fenster). Barth, Leipzig, 1958.

28. Livingston, W.K. Pain mechanisms. A physiological interpretation of causalgia and its related states. Macmillan, New York, 1943, unabridged version published by Plenum Press (1976).

29. Loh, L., Nathan, P.W., Schott, G.D., Wilson, P.G. Effects of regional guanethidine infusion in certain painful states. J Neurol Neurosurg Psychiatry, 43: 446-451, 1980.

30. Maurer, G. Umbau, Dystrophy und Atrophie an den Gliedmaßen. (Sogennannte Sudeck'sche Knochenatrophie). Ergeb Chirurg, 33: 476-531, 1941.

31. Mellander, S., Johansson, B.   Control of resistance exchange and capacitance functions in the peripheral circulation. Pharmacol Rev, 20: 117-196, 1968.

32. Mittelmeier, H., Biehl, G. Sudeck-Syndrome. In: Witt, A.N., Rettig, H., Schlegel, K.F., Hackenbroch, M., Hupfauer, W. (Hrsg.), Orthopadie in Praxis und Klinik, Thieme, Stuttgart, pp. 8.1-8.13, 1982.

33. Morsier, G.   Les troubles reflexes consécutifs aux traumatismes des membres. Schweiz Arch Neurol Psychiat, 59: 239-317, 1947.

34. Moskowitz, E., Bishop, H.F., Shibutani, K.   Posthemiplegic reflex sympathetic dystrophy. JAMA, 167: 836-838, 1958.

35. Nathan, P.W.   On the pathogenesis of causalgia in peripheral nerve injuries. Brain, 70: 145-170, 1947.

36. Pak, T.J., Martin, G.M., Magness, J.L., Kavanaugh, G.J.   Reflex sympathetic dystrophy. Minn Med: 507-512, 1970.

37. Patman, R.D., Thompson, J.E., Persson, A.V.   Management of post-traumatic pain syndromes: Report of 113 cases. Ann Surg, 177: 780-787, 1973.

38. Rasmussen, T.B., Freedman, H. Treatment of causalgia. J Neurosurg, 3: 165-173, 1946.

39. Roberts, W.J. A hypothesis on the physiological basis for causalgia and related pains. Pain, 24: 297-311, 1986.

40. Rowell, L.B.   Cardiovascular adjustments to thermal stress. In: J.T. Shepherd, F.M. Abboud, S.R. Geiger, (Eds.), Handbook of Physiology, Section 2: The Cardiovascular System, Vol. III, pp. 967-1023, 1983.

41. Schwartzman, R.J., McLellan, T.L. Reflex sympathetic dystrophy. Arch Neurol, 44: 555-561, 1987.

42. Shumacker, H.B. Causalgia. Surgery, 24: 458-504, 1948.

43. Steinbrocker, O., Spitzer, N., Friedman, H. The shoulder-hand syndrome in reflex dystrophy of the upper extremity. Ann Intern Med, 29: 22-52, 1948.

44. Sudeck, P. Ueber die akute (trophoneurotische) Knochenatrophie nach Entzündungen und Traumen der Extremitäten. Dtsch Med Wochenschr, 28: 336-338, 1902.

45. Sudeck, P. Kollaterale Entzundungszustande, sog.akute Knochenatrophie und Dystrophie der Gliedmassen in der Unfallheilkunde. Vogel, Berlin, 1938.

46. Sudeck, P. Die sogen. akute Knochenatrophie als Entzundungsvorgang. Chirurg, 14: 449-458, 1942.

47. Sunderland, S. Pain mechanisms in causalgia. J Neurol Neurosurg Psychiatry, 39: 471-480, 1976.

48. Thompson, M. Shoulder-hand syndrome. Proc Soc Med, 54: 679-684, 1961.

49. Thorban, W. Klinische und experimentelle Untersuchungen zur Ätiologie und Pathogenese der posttraumatischen Sudeckschen GliedmaBendystrophie. Acta Neuroveg, 25: 1-62, 1962.

50. Trostdorf, E. Die Kausalgie. Thieme, Stuttgart, 1956.

51. Winter, S. Sympathetic reflex dystrophies in coronary heart disease. NY State J Med, 54: 2330-2332, 1954.

52. Witzleb, E. Funktionen des GefäBsystems. In: R. F. Schmidt, G. Thews (Eds.), Physiologie des Menschen. Springer, Berlin, pp. 434-498, 1985.

SUMMARY OF SECTION II

BASIC RESEARCHES IN PATHOPHYSIOLOGY OF RSD

The discussion first focused on the causes of edema formation in reflex sympathetic dystrophy. It was stated that the underlying imbalance between pre- and postcapillary pressures need not be the result of a difference in sympathetic constrictor tone between arterioloes and venules; it also could be caused by a differential sensitivity of arterial and venous vascular muscle to the same sympathetic activity. Hypoxia and other local metabolic processes could also be a cause. In addition, vasoactive substances released from nociceptors intensify vascular permeability. Nevertheless, sympathetic malfunction is present and can be demonstrated by abnormal thermoregulatory responses in the affected area.

It was stated that the tissue pressure caused by the edema may in fact be the cause of spontaneous pain: in bone and deep solid tissues like palms or soles the edema cannot expand and a pressure high enough to stimulate nociceptors may be the result. This is consistent with the clinical observation that pain is alleviated by reducing hydrostatic pressure (i.e., lifting hand or foot). In case of sensitized nociceptors even small pressure increases may be sufficient to produce pain.

However, spontaneous pain is not merely caused by nociceptor activity; together with allodynia it may be the result of abnormal processing of information from low threshold mechano- or thermoreceptors by spinal multireceptive neurones (i.e., convergent or WDR neurones). Further evidence for the underlying central dysfunction coming from reaction time studies in patients with mechanical and/or thermal allodynia were cited: reaction times to innocuous tactile, cold or warm pulses on the abnormal side were modality specific and did not differ from those on the normal side. This suggests that the afferent impulses which elicit pain, originate from low threshold mechano, cold and warm receptors, respective.

Overall, this was an enlightening session which helped develop new ideas and concepts regarding the pathophysiological processed mediating the syndrome of reflex sympathetic dystrophy.

Section III

THERAPEUTIC TECHNIQUES IN RSD

11

SYMPATHETIC NERVE BLOCKS: Their role in sympathetic pain

Robert A. Boas

Selective and complete sympathetic block with local anesthetic or neurolytic agents, requires that solution be placed at the sympathetic chain in such a way as to avoid other surrounding structures. Standard approaches as described by Bonica (1) and Moore (2), use anatomical landmarks and tactile control, promoting high but not perfect success rates. However, in pain management, and especially in those cases receiving neurolytic injection, it is important that no extraneous solution spreads to involve other nerves or structures. Selective, safe and functionally distinct sympathetic block, at either cervical or lumbar levels, is best performed by means of fluoroscopic radiological screening of both needle placement and subsequent solution injection. This is probably not necessary for out patient based stellate blocks, where convenience, simplicity, and economy allow use of high volume local anesthetic procedures without undue concern for long-term risks of aberrant spread. However, when nerve destruction is sought utilising neurolytic, cryogenic, or radiofrequency lesions, then X-ray screening should be mandatory.

SYMPATHETIC BLOCKS AS AN AID
TO DIAGNOSIS IN RSD

In this context, Reflex Sympathetic Dystrophy (RSD) is defined as a symptom complex or syndrome, presenting with diffuse, distal nonsegmental, burning pain in a limb following local trauma or disease. Hallmarks of the dystrophic state as opposed to other neuropathies, include allodynia and a characteristic adoptive posture seeking to provide stimulus protection. Included are the autonomic, motor and sensory signs, as described by Blumberg et al. in the previous chapter, and summarised in the appendix of this text. Provocation of pain by cold stimulation can be used as a confirmatory test (3), as can radionuclide bone scanning (4). The most specific confirmatory test is a positive response following sympathetic block. Post block changes should be evident within a few minutes, exhibiting reversal of sympathetic effector responses and return of normal cutaneous sensation. Mere reduction in pain or removal of only one component to the painful symptom complex, usually signifies an effector component contributing to or maintaining part of the pain. This would constitute a state of sympathetically maintained pain in a more circumscribed and sustained local disorder. But when pain is abolished and other criteria are also satisfied as discussed by Wilson in Chapter 4, then the condition is truly one of a sympathetic dystrophy. Importance in making this strong distinction lies in subsequent emphasis given to therapies aimed at resolution of differing underlying pathologies.

This same post-block evaluation process gives opportunity for separation of underlying somatic pain from the symptom complex. Somatic pain is unaffected by efferent blockade, though peripheral neuropathic and perhaps some other pain states may be sensitised by local noradrenaline release (5). Sustained nociceptive input from a somatic focus of disease or injury is often the stimulus initiating a reflex cycle, but because sympathetic dystrophy pain so overwhelms, identification of primary lesions is not always possible. Long-term resolution of the symptom complex, almost always requires that therapy be directed at both the primary lesion as well as the secondary dystrophy. Diagnostic criteria and the role of sympathetic blocks can therefore be presented as follows.

Etiology. Local trauma or painful unresolved disease. Passive or non-use posture of limb.

Symptoms. Diffuse burning nonsegmental limb pain.

Signs. Cold, sweating, dusky limb colouration. Trophic changes in skin, nails and hair. Swelling, weakness and joint stiffness in the limb. Proximal spread and symptomatic progression with time.

Tests. Sympathetic block or regional adrenergic blockade abolishes symptoms and efferent sympathetic activity. Increased ipsilateral vasoconstriction to cold stress. Pain provocation with cold. Distinctive radionuclide screening pattern.

While RSD is a generic term describing painful disorders with some or all of these features, several descriptive terms of long traditional use have been retained in the literature. They differ only in the primary lesion, subsequent progression to RSD being similar in each.

MANAGEMENT PRINCIPLES FOR RSD
AND SYMPATHETIC BLOCK USE

Perhaps the most important point bearing emphasis is for patients to take greater responsibility for their own care. Because disuse and loss of normal sensory input appear to play such an important part in pathogenesis of the dystrophic state, so too must activity be resumed in order to sustain relief and ultimate resolution. Sympathetic block merely interrupts the cycle, thereby facilitating the return of activity, normal sensory input and venous outflow as proposed by Blumberg and others above. Patients should be encouraged to make full use of pain free periods to undertake physical exercise as the definitive therapy for RSD. Exercises should be active, regular and gentle until such time as strength and mobility return. Activity should be pursued to the point of obsession, "several minutes on the hour, every hour," being an admonition which seems to deliver the message. Reliance on sympathetic block alone may therefore be insufficient to achieve a lasting cure, especially in cases with secondary joint, ligamentous, muscle and trophic changes causing addition pain on exercise. For such cases somatic nerve block may provide a more complete relief of pain and allow for better exercise therapy, provided the block does not also induce motor paralysis (see Raj et al., Chapter 17). In every case, the underlying cause for the RSD must also be resolved, or a dystrophy may well recur.

REGIONAL BLOCKS

The frequency with which repeat local anesthetic blocks are undertaken may be twice weekly or more, declining as improvement progresses to become weekly, then biweekly until relief is sustained and exercise maintains symptomatic remission. When exercise is still painful even after block, a focus to additional pain sites may be needed with other therapies. Transcutaneous electrical stimulation, focal steroid injections, repair of remedial lesions or symptomatic analgesic cover, may be appropriate. Sometimes responses are dramatic and complete, but long-standing cases with advanced trophic changes or joint restriction, or those with underlying painful lesions, may take several months of vigorous therapy and many blocks in order to bring about resolution.

PSYCHOTHERAPY

For those clinicians who feel that psychosomatic factors play a part in the etiology of RSD, the literature is conflicting, as the papers in this text demonstrate. What is usually evident is the anxious, passive, defensive and protective behaviour which so many patients display. There should in such cases, be a more structured analysis of patient's problems and fears which may then reveal features amenable to additional counselling and treatment. It may be difficult to gain a patient's confidence and cooperation to conduct block procedures without also addressing their fears and anxieties, as presented by Haddox in this text.

MEDICATIONS as adjunctive therapy

Combined therapies are the rule rather than the exception for treatment of most resistant cases, as exemplified in Chapter 17. At the least, small night doses of tricyclic antidepressants can help bring about sleep improvement and reduction in primary neuropathic pain if that is a factor, irrespective of any accompanying depressive tendencies. Opiate analgesics are ineffective in suppression of RSD pains. They should be withdrawn gradually as part of therapy if already initiated, as they appear to sustain the central component of neuronal hyperactivity, promote drug dependence and constrain self-reliance. See Chapter 3 for detailed guidance. Some conditions respond to steroids, either as part of an anti-inflammatory action or as membrane stabilising drugs when applied directly to damaged nerves (6). Yet others without focal responsiveness, show apparent systemic benefits to oral steroid therapy in well controlled studies, to the point of resolution (7). Whether other membrane stabilisers, such as beta blockers and calcium antagonists, have a place is essentially untried (8), the topic of this and ancillary therapies being well reviewed by Charlton in Chapter 19. On the other hand, some evidence for benefit does exist for efferent adrenergic blockade, whether at the level of nerve conduction block, peripheral transmitter release or post junctional receptor blockade, as already reviewed. Where allodynia prevents use of a pressure tourniquet or access to an intravenous site for a guanethidine block, then a regional local anesthetic ganglion block is the first treatment of choice.

To summarise thus far, several points are reiterated.

1. Exercise is fundamental to symptomatic and functional improvement.
2. Sympathetic or noradrenergic blockade provides symptomatic benefit to allow exercise therapy.
3. Treatment may be needed for concurrent underlying disease.
4. Psychogenic factors are not primary to RSD.
5. Patients need counselling with recognition of their own pivotal role in gaining resolution.
6. Analgesic medications are ineffective for RSD pain therapy.

TECHNIQUES OF SYMPATHETIC BLOCK

Stellate Block

Classical approaches to cervico-thoracic (stellate) sympathetic blocks are well described in the texts already cited. There have been no procedural advances since, the only points of contention being whether needle insertion should be directed to the 6th or 7th cervical level. Each has advantages, C6 for lessened risk of pneumothorax and C7 for greater certainty of blocking sympathetics to the arm. In either case, common risks of inadvertent vascular injection or subdural root sleeve puncture, can be lessened by the use of extension tubing between the injecting needle and aspirating syringe. An assistant is required to make frequent aspirations intermittently during needle insertion and subsequent injection of local anaesthetic. Close patient observation provides the other critical safeguard. C7 needle placement promotes a more caudad solution spread with small volumes, reaching superior and inferior thoracic ganglia (9), giving more complete sympathetic block to the arm. Patients should be fully conscious during stellate blocks to allow for careful observation, monitoring and reporting of adverse responses.

LUMBAR SYMPATHETIC BLOCK

Single needle approaches, with patients prone or lying on their side and with placement at either L2 or L3, provide effective physiological and functional block (10). Use of an 8-10cm approach from the midline allows for ready access to the antero-lateral margin of vertebral bodies at the site of the sympathetic chain and its ganglia. If a more sagittal insertion plane is employed, solution spreads more laterally into psoas sheath, with greater risk of genito-femoral nerve injury. Even so, some prefer this median approach because needle penetration through the kidney is less frequent. There is, however, no evidence that this carries any risk, although ureteric necrosis is described using nonscreened neurolytic block.

In some cases, despite apparent accurate needle placement, it is difficult if not impossible to obtain correct solution spread in the tissue plane containing sympathetic fibres. Increasing the volume of injectate merely disseminates abnormal spread. While this may be acceptable with local anaesthetic, neurolytic injection is safer when the chain is sought again at another level. Correctly placed, volumes in the order of 10-15 ml are usually adequate to achieve spread over two segmental levels with a single needle, as is shown in Figure 1.

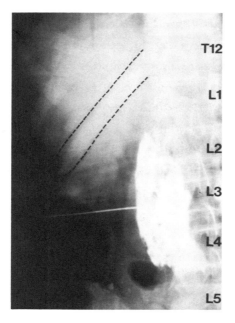

Figure 1. Radiographic depiction of phenol spread with 8ml of solution injected at L3 level with a single needle technique. Note confinement of spread within medial limits of psoas and longitudinal extension over three segmental levels when correctly placed at the lumbar sympathetic chain.

DRUG CHOICE

Choice of local anesthetic agents is not important. Once block is established, symptomatic improvement outlasts drug action itself, so choice concerns are directed to potential aberrant spread or drug toxicity. For these reasons, shorter acting agents such as lidocaine or prilocaine offer quick onset and greater safety, and are recommended. Neurolytic agents include alcohol 50-100% or phenol 6-12%, either in water or a radio-opaque contrast solution. The literature is almost devoid of reports using alcohol for other than celiac plexus block, perhaps because it is so painful, but also because of fears relating to extraneous injections. Phenol injections in contrast solutions are stable and safe, having withstood more than 10 years of use and many thousand injections without consequence since first report (11). Studies by Gregg et al. (12) indicate however, that regeneration of all nerve fibres occurs over a matter of weeks, and that even 12% solutions may provide only extended rather than permanent blockade (Figure 2). Higher concentrations gave somewhat more complete and sustained effects, suggesting 10% or 12% solutions should be employed as routine. Further dose response relationships or duration studies afford an excellent opportunity for important clinical research. Neurolytic stellate blocks are rarely used because of the serious risks involved, but with proper technique this is probably only of theoretical concern. Certainly at a lumbar level it is practice to use phenol, in other than children or adolescents, because it obviates the need for repeat procedures. Preference for guanethidine blocks, in other than the first week or two, has also displaced repeat stellate ganglion blocks in some practice.

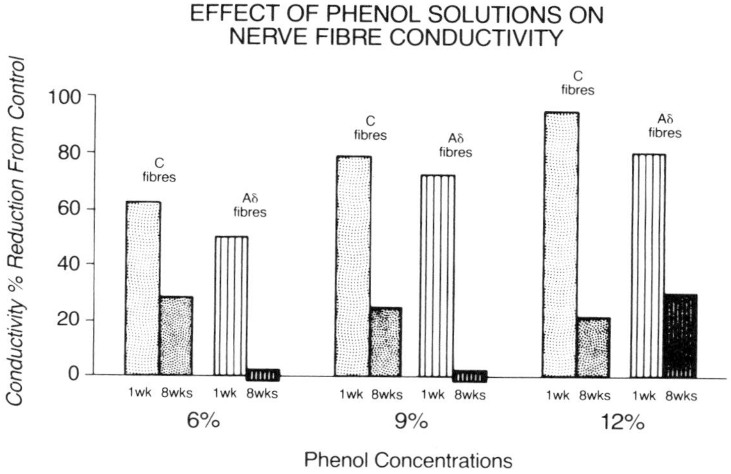

EFFECT OF PHENOL SOLUTIONS ON
NERVE FIBRE CONDUCTIVITY

Figure 2.   Neurolytic action of phenol in renographin is greater with increasing concentrations of phenol, irrespective of the fibre type or size. Spontaneous regeneration occurs rapidly and functional return is almost complete after 8 weeks in all fibres. Derived from Gregg et al., 1985 (12).

ASSESSMENT

A multiplicity of tests have been reported as objective scalar measures of response to sympathetic block. Lofstrom and Cousins (13) in their review provide extensive discussion on twenty-two such tests. Perhaps the simplest, cheapest and most convenient is thermistor cutaneous temperature monitoring. Following sympathetic block for RSD, changes of 5-10°C are the norm, but reflect only part of the responses to efferent interruption.   Sweat testing is probably more specific to RSD, and may provide a tool for comparative research studies.   Indices of several features common to dystrophic changes have also been proposed, but in the clinical context documentation of pain, temperature, color, sweating, strength and range of motion changes, are probably adequate for patient follow-up.

Practical features can be summarised briefly:

1. Complete reliability of block performance requires X-ray monitoring.
2. Careful observation and patient monitoring is always required.
3. Neurolytic blocks should incorporate a contrast solution.
4. Results should be documented by objective changes.

RESULTS OF SYMPATHETIC BLOCK TREATMENT FOR RSD

Despite an extensive 50 year literature on the subject, there is a paucity of properly conducted trials on sympathetic block use for RSD. This seems perhaps a raison d'etre for this workshop, and may help provoke further clinical studies on the subject. Be that as it may, anecdotal reports abound, most advocating similar philosophies to those expounded above. One comparative randomised study found little long-term difference between guanethidine or sympathetic block (14) while another retrospective report showed a significantly better outcome with block as against more conservative therapies (15). All reports describe refractory cases, but none give a comprehensive three part management approach as advocated above (**blocks-exercise-local treatments**), though a review by Schutzer et al. (16) contains a well balanced and experienced concept of management. So many therapists follow a unitary narrowly defined specialty approach to care, that a lead should be taken by multidisciplinary pain groups to establish a sounder and substantiated basis to RSD treatment.

CONCLUSIONS

Anatomical and procedural details for the conduct of sympathetic blocks could fill several chapters, but the scientific presentation of well controlled outcome studies barely allows for a paragraph. Our relative ignorance of pathophysiological mechanisms may account in part for this deficiency, though the tools for better clinical measurements and outcome audits are probably available to all. Since no controlled prospective studies have yet been reported, this would seem a fertile area for multicenter trials. Agreement on details of diagnostic criteria, treatment and response measurement protocols, seem minor obstacles for what could be rewarding clinical research. This volume and its ultimate consensus, should help achieve such studies.

REFERENCES

1. Bonica, J.J. Management of pain. Philadelphia, Lea and Febiger, 1953.
2. Moore, D.C. Stellate ganglion block. Springfield, Thomas, 1954.
3. Frost, S.A., Raja, S.N., Campbell, J.N., Meyer, R.A., Khan, A.A. Does hyperalgesia to cooling stimuli characterise patients with sympathetically maintained pain (Reflex Sympathetic Dystrophy)? Proceedings of the 5th World Congress on Pain. Editors: Dubner, R., Gebhart, G.F., Bond, M.R. Amsterdam, Elsevier, pp. 151-156, 1988.
4. Holder, L.E., Mackinnon, S.E. Reflex sympathetic dystrophy in the hands: Clinical and scintigraphic criteria. Radiology, 152, 2: 517-522, 1984.
5. Wall, P.D., Gutnick, M. Ongoing activity in peripheral nerves: The physiology and pharmacology of impulses originating from a neuroma. Exp. Neurol., 43: 580-593, 1974.
6. Devor, M., Govrin-Lippmann, R., Raber, P. Corticosteroids suppress ectopic neural discharge originating in experimental neuromas. Pain, 22: 127-137, 1985.
7. Christensen, K., Jensen, E.M., Noer, I. The reflex dystrophy syndrome response to treatment with systemic corticosteroids. Acta Chir. Scand., 148: 653-655, 1982.
8. Plough, 1985.
9. Boas, R.A., Hatangdi, V.S. Chemical sympathectomy - techniques and responses. In Yokota, T., Dubner, R. (eds.), Current topics in pain research and therapy. Amsterdam, Excerpta Medica, pp. 259-269, 1983.
10. Hatangdi, V.S., Boas, R.A. Lumbar sympathectomy: A single needle technique. Brit. J. Anaesth., 57: 285-289, 1985.

11. Boas, R.A., Hatangdi, V.S., Richards, E.G. Lumbar sympathectomy, a percutaneous chemical technique. In Bonica, J.J., Albe-Fessard, D. (eds.), Advances in pain research and therapy, vol. 1. New York, Raven Press, pp. 685-689, 1976.

12. Gregg, R.V., Constantin, C.H., Ford, D.J., Raj, P.P., Means, E. Electrophysiologic and histopathologic investigation of phenol in renographin as a neurolytic agent. Anesthesiology, 63: 31, A239, 1985.

13. Lofstrom, B.J., Cousins, M.J. Sympathetic neural blockade of the upper and lower extremity. In Cousins, M.J., Breidenbaugh, P.O. (eds.), Neural blockade, 2nd ed. Philadelphia, J.B. Lippincott Co., pp. 461-500, 1988.

14. Bonelli, S., Conoscente, F., Movilia, P.G., Restelli, L., Francucci, B., Grossi, E. Regional intravenous guanethidine vs. stellate ganglion block in reflex sympathetic dystrophies: A randomised trial. Pain, 16: 297-307, 1983.

15. Wang, J.K., Johnson, K.E., Ilstrup, D.M. Sympathetic blocks for reflex sympathetic dystrophy. Pain, 23: 13-17, 1985.

16. Schutzer, S.F., Gossling, H.R., Connecticut, F. The treatment of reflex sympathetic dystrophy syndrome. J. Bone and Joint Surg., 66-1, 4: 625-629, 1984.

12

INTRAVENOUS REGIONAL SYMPATHETIC BLOCKS

Dr. J. G. Hannington-Kiff

The introduction of intravenous regional guanethidine (IVRG) block in 1974 (1,2) has transformed the management of reflex sympathetic dystrophy (RSD). This successful technique has notably withstood the test of time, and remains one of the most effective ways of treating limbs (especially the hands) disabled by RSD. Moreover, the guanethidine technique has generated many new ideas about the etiology of this enigmatic condition (3). The main limitation of the guanethidine technique on a world-wide basis is the unavailability of parenteral guanethidine in some countries. Reserpine and bretylium have a similar action to guanethidine, and can be used as substitutes in the IVR technique but their effects are less clinically useful. Alpha-adrenoceptor blockers such as thymoxamine can be used in the IVR technique to produce antisympathetic block but again the results are poor compared with guanethidine.

The principle of the guanethidine technique is that a very high concentration of the drug can be applied directly to the sympathetic nerve endings in the treated extremity, producing a noradrenergic neuron block. The sympathetic nerve endings rewardingly assist the process by avidly taking up the guanethidine. It is important to realize that the sympathetic nerve endings have a natural mechanism--the amine uptake pump--which recovers much of the noradrenaline (NA) after its secretion into the junctional cleft. This is a characteristic of noradrenergic neurons in contrast with cholinergic neurons. After secretion, acetylcholine is rapidly broken down in the junctional cleft by cholinesterase, so the nerves must continuously produce acetylcholine.

Sympathetic nerve endings are unable to distinguish guanethidine from NA so therefore the amine uptake pump causes noradrenergic neurons to accumulate guanethidine. Since guanethidine now occupies the NA storage sites, the sympathetic nerve endings are unable to replenish their NA stores. The overall effect is a noradrenergic (sympathetic) block. The presence of guanethidine in the sympathetic nerve endings also reduces the action potential and interferes with the release of NA. It has been shown experimentally that guanethidine can actually damage the noradrenergic neurons in a number of ways. The amine uptake pump can be chronically reduced in efficiency, axon transport can be adversely affected, the nerves can be damaged or destroyed by a kind of autoimmune reaction and the curious phenomenon of axon retraction can occur. Following axon retraction there is an increased gap between the sympathetic nerve ending and the receptor site thus weakening the effect of the released NA. Consequently, there are possibilities both for functional and for structural sympathectomy confined to the treated limb.

COMPARISON WITH SYMPATHETIC GANGLION BLOCK

The established method of temporarily blocking the regional sympathetic nerve supply to a limb is the injection of local anesthetic agent into the stellate ganglion or the thoraco-lumbar ganglion-chain supplying the arm and leg, respectively. The prime indication for the IVRG block is in the upper extremity. The IVRG block is more difficult to perform in the lower limb because of the greater mass and circumference of the limb, the greater technical problems, and the extra hazards associated with the tourniquet and the more difficult cannulation of veins. Moreover, the lumbar ganglion block is so easy, accurate and uncomplicated with the aid of image-intensified x-ray control that it is preferable to the IVRG block in the leg and foot.

It is notable that sympathetic ganglion block with local anesthesia interrupts both noradrenergic and cholinergic nerve fibres whereas IVRG block only affects the noradrenergic nerve fibres. Consequently, the ganglion block will stop sweating in the treated limb clinically relevant? If the patient has a troublesome sweaty palm or sole, a ganglion block will cause drying whereas sweating will be unaffected by the IVRG block because sudomotor activity is cholinergic. It should be noted that some moisture on the palm is necessary for a good grip so that the artisan being treated for RSD may be better served by IVRG blocks if the affected hand can still be used to some extent.

THE IVRG BLOCK

A reliable tourniquet is essential. Uniform pressure has to be applied to the limb for 20 minutes with the least discomfort for the patient. The pressure must exceed the systolic pressure by a minimum of 50 mm and 100 mm Hg in the upper and lower limb, respectively. Higher excess pressures than these are preferable because the patient will, on the whole, suffer less discomfort from a high tourniquet pressure than a lower one which allows the treated limb to swell by the ingress of arterial blood. The combined effects of the seepage of arterial blood into the limb and the injected volume of dilute guanethidine solution may so raise the pressure in the veins that the tourniquet will allow guanethidine to enter the general circulation before it is fixed in the tissues.

The dose of guanethidine should not exceed 30mg in any single block, or 150 mg guanethidine in any course of treatment. If the patient does not respond after 5-6 IVRG blocks, ganglion blocks and other strategies should be employed. The initial IVRG block in RSD should be limited to 10 mg because these patients have a high incidence of Raynaud-type reactivity of the peripheral circulation which predisposes them to increased vasoconstriction in response to the marked release of NA by the first use of guanethidine. In subsequent blocks, repeated within 3-5 days, the dose of guanethidine can be increased as the sympathetic nerve endings become "tamed" by the cumulative effect of guanethidine so that there is less release of NA.

The dose of guanethidine should also be adjusted according to the size of the limb (the upper limb being smaller than the lower limb), and according to the general physical state of the patient. The dose of guanethidine can be reduced by applying the tourniquet more distally on the limb, or by the use of a second more distal venous occlusion tourniquet as well. The volume of physiological saline in which the guanethidine solution is diluted should be commensurate with the volume of the limb to be treated. As a general guide the volume of saline used in the upper and lower limbs with the tourniquet on the upper arm or thigh would be about 25 ml and 50 ml, respectively. It should be borne in the mind that higher dilution of the guanethidine solution can reduce the strength of the block.

Interactions of Guanethidine

Guanethidine is a strongly basic substance and consideration should be given to the possible in vitro interaction between guanethidine and other agents mixed with it in solution. Heparin (strongly acidic) was mixed with guanethidine when the technique was first introduced (1,2) but this has proved unnecessary in practice and was soon abandoned in the IVRG technique. It is common practice to mix a local anesthetic agent with the dilute guanethidine solution, causing no chemical interaction. Now that prilocaine is widely advocated as the safest agent for IVR anaesthesia, only the preservative-free solution specially made for this purpose should be used. The methylhydroxybenzoated preservative can cause some pain and irritation (4). Before performing an IVRG block, it should be established whether the patient is taking any prescribed medicines or misusing any substances which could interact with the guanethidine. For example, the patient on a monoamine oxidase inhibitor, accumulates NA in the sympathetic nerves so that a dose of guanethidine could cause a relatively high release of NA and precipitate a hypertensive crisis. Sympathomimetic drugs and tricyclic antidepressants interfere with the uptake of guanethidine by the sympathetic nerve endings so that the blocking effect of the guanethidine may be less. When the patient is being treated with a course of IVRG blocks, he should be warned about taking direct acting sympathomimetic agents which can result in hypertension and dysrhythmia.

ADVANTAGES OF THE IVRG BLOCK

Simplicity

One of the prime advantages of the IVRG technique of blocking the sympathetic nervous system is that the only expertise required is the ability to cannulate a vein, whereas sympathetic ganglion blocks require a degree of skill not possessed by most doctors. Herein, paradoxically, there lies some danger because it is important that well informed care be used in application of the tourniquet to ensure maximum safety.

Duration and Repetition

An IVRG block may be expected to last with obvious clinical antisympathetic effect for 2-3 days compared with a few hours after local anaesthetic ganglion block. The duration of IVRG block becomes longer after frequent repetition because guanethidine accumulates in the sympathetic nerves and causes progressive functional and structural damage.

IVRG blocks can be repeated at short intervals with little distress to the patient, but it is necessary to regard the IVRG technique as a facilitatory maneuver, assisting in promotion of re-use of the limb affected by RSD. The initial relief of pain and disability must be capitalized upon by the energetic use of physical measures which reinforce and establish the functional rehabilitation of the limb, as emphasized in the previous chapter by Boas.

Research

Guanethidine produces a profound and total blocking effect on the sympathetic nerve endings by uncoupling pharmacological mechanisms associated with the release of NA, ATP (adenosine triphosphate) and NPY (neuropeptide Y), all of which can affect the tone of vascular smooth muscle. The appropriate consecutive use of other antagonistic drugs could be used in the IVR technique in an attempt to determine whether other consequences of RSD are caused by triggers other than NA. For example, the IVR use of a calcium channel blocker such as verapamil could be used to determine whether ATP was the trigger of pain and disability in a dystrophic limb. (ATP is electromechanically released by the action of calcium ions).

Other possibilities are the use of ketanserin to block the effect of 5-HT (5-hydroxytryptamine), lysine acetylsalicylate to block prostaglandins and naftidrofuryl (Praxiline) to block bradykinin. Clearly the IVR technique may be a powerful research tool in RSD.

There are similarities between RSD and the early stages of rheumatoid arthritis. The use of IVRG blocks has also proved useful in palindromic rheumatism (5) and in dealing with exacerbations of pain and loss of function in established rheumatoid arthritis (6).

DISADVANTAGES OF IVRG BLOCK

Extra Equipment

Compared with the stellate ganglion block, which basically requires a syringe and needle, the need for exsanguination of the limb and the use of a tourniquet, make the guanethidine block more time consuming. In the case of lumbar sympathetic ganglion block, during which X-ray control with an image intensifier should be mandatory, there is little to choose between ganglion block and IVR technique with regard to expediency.

Tourniquet Failure

This is the main cause for concern with the IVR technique. Paradoxically, the very simplicity of the IVRG block may tempt an uninformed beginner to undertake the method. The IVRG block should only be used (as with ganglion blocks) by experienced personnel, in a clinic environment, with full resuscitation facilities. Accidents can happen even in skilled hands.

If the limb is carefully observed during the performance of IVRG block, the skin will first be seen to become irregularly blotchy with pale central zones surrounded by livid edges. This is probably the result of arteriolar constriction caused by the initial release of NA by guanethidine. This supposition is supported by the concurrent complaint of stinging (causalgic) pain by the RSD patient. This stage of NA release lasts from 5-7 minutes, making it theoretically possible that tourniquet failure at this early stage could cause a rapid rise in blood pressure, owing to release of unfixed NA into the circulation. In practice, the fall of blood pressure after planned tourniquet release at about 20 minutes is minimal and clinically insignificant provided the patient is at rest.

Discomfort

The application of a tourniquet to a painful limb is sometimes intolerable for the patient and a regional block more proximally, or a general anesthetic is required. To avert pain on guanethidine injection, a local anesthetic IVR can be used preemptively. During the course of subsequent treatments, the alleviation of discomfort is usually progressive, and the need for these other measures becomes less or unnecessary. Much of the average patient's intolerance of the IVR technique is caused by unfamiliarity with the procedure, and it is common for patients to tolerate repeat blocks with equanimity.

Two tips may be given. First, unless the patient has quite severe limb pain and can obviously not tolerate the tourniquet without assistance, only the smallest amount of intravenous sedation with diazepam should be given, perhaps supplemented with 50:50 nitrous oxide and oxygen inhalation. Otherwise the patient may become dis-inhibited to the point of being unmanageable. Second, a tight tourniquet can paradoxically be more bearable than the situation in which the tourniquet allows a slight leak of arterial blood into the limb with subsequent swelling and seepage of guanethidine into the general circulation. Therefore, it is not only unwise to choose a marginal difference between the systolic arterial pressure and the tourniquet pressure, but any hope that the lower tourniquet pressure is more tolerable for the patient may well be unfounded.

Minor Complications

It is common practice to add a small amount of local anesthetic to the guanethidine solution before its injection, because of the exacerbation of pain caused by the initial release of NA by the guanethidine. Prilocaine without preservative is a good choice for this purpose (4). The release of NA by subsequent blocks should be less if the blocks are repeated at intervals of under 5 days. For this reason, and because the patient's pain should have responded to overall treatment, there should be no need for the inclusion of local anesthetic in repeat blocks.

Some patients complain of a dry throat and a light-heated feeling just after release of the tourniquet. The eyes may become slightly dry, the conjunctivae pink and the upper lids may droop for a short time. Some patients mention that they feel drowsy and floppy (possibly because of muscle weakness) for up to a couple of days after an IVRG block. These effects are rather nonspecific any may reflect, in part, the relative relaxation that must accompany the relief of pain following the guanethidine block. Moreover, in clinical practice patients commonly receive other drugs such as intravenous diazepam in association with the guanethidine block and the precise attribution of the side effects can be difficult.

*Note. In subsequent discussion it became evident that others had experiences with post-block episodes of postural hypotension, particularly with frequent repeat guanethidine blocks, or in cases using 30mg doses.

Reports of diarrhea for one to two days following block, were also evident. (Eds)

Drug Interactions

The patient should be asked about current medication because some drugs can interact adversely with guanethidine. Amongst prescribed drugs the main categories that may preclude the use of IVRG blocks are monoamine oxidase inhibitors, tricyclic antidepressants and various amphetamine-like drugs. It should be routine to ask patients whether they are taking any non-prescription drugs, amphetamine-like drugs for slimming, alertness, etc., or whether they are using sympathomimetic drugs. Caution is required with certain other categories of drugs such as antihypertensive agents, and the manufacturer's data sheet should be consulted for full details.

SPECIAL INDICATIONS

Occasionally, it is not feasible to produce sympathetic block by injecting the regional paravertebral ganglia and it was for this reason that the IVRG technique was first introduced. The following are the main special indications for IVRG block.

Bleeding Tendency

Paravertebral ganglion blocks are hazardous in patients taking anticoagulants and in patients with bleeding disorders. Under these circumstances a block requiring only venepuncture should be uneventful.

Scar Tissue

Scar tissue or cancer infiltration in the vicinity of the regional paravertebral ganglia can make local anesthetic block difficult with unreliable results. Similarly, if a neurolytic solution has been injected into the ganglia previously (as in the lumbar region), then adhesions and scarring, predisposing to poor response with a regional local anesthetic block, will be more likely.

Failed Sympathectomy

Sympathetic tone can reappear in a limb a few months after seemingly adequate surgical sympathectomy, and there may be recrudescence of the previous symptoms and signs of RSD. In this situation the IVRG technique is still effective in producing regional sympathetic block, which may be effective for as long as 3 months.

Localized Vasodilatation

The profound vasodilatation of IVRG block is confirmed to a selected part of a limb rather than affecting a quadrant of the body as happens after a ganglion block. This can be exploited by the use of IVRG block confined by a tourniquet at the wrist or a band round the digit, in replantation surgery. Such mini-IVRG blocks might also be useful in the detailed investigation of RSD confined to one or more fingers.

Direct Guanethidine Effect

Guanethidine has a direct relaxant effect on vascular smooth muscle in addition to the vasodilating effect of the regional noradrenergic nerve block which it produces. This could be useful in improving the blood supply to striated muscle, which is mainly under direct control by "chemical" changes in the blood flowing through the muscle. Ganglion blocks are known to favor an increase in skin blood flow, which can "steal" blood flow from muscle in ischemic limbs. It is possible that this "steal phenomenon" is less after the IVRG technique.

Finally, a remarkable reduction in high-turnover osteoporosis (as shown by radionuclide scanning), can occur in the bone of limbs affected by RSD following only one guanethidine block (7). This change also occurs after sympathetic ganglion block but is not so profound in degree. Is it possible that the guanethidine has a direct beneficial effect on the osteoblasts, having been delivered there by the nutrient vessels of the bone?

CLINICAL STRATEGY

Early Treatment

Early diagnosis, early referral and early treatment are the keys to success in the management of RSD. The profusion of diagnostic labels applied to RSD has inhibited its early recognition. Though it is not that uncommon, RSD usually only merits a mention in most orthopaedic textbooks, where it is more often referred to as Sudeck's strophy. In these texts, so much emphasis is attached to the X-ray finding of osteoporosis, that RSD is diagnosed relatively late when this feature is obvious. For osteoporosis to be evident on routine radiographs, 35% of the bone must have been absorbed. The diagnosis of RSD should be a clinical one, based upon the criteria presented in Chapter 4 by Wilson.

Patients often recognize early on, that a minor injury has become complicated by inappropriate pain and disability. These patients are frequently dismissed as neurotic until the signs of RSD are well advanced.

Team Approach

It is important to accept that the IVRG block is only one step up the ladder towards rehabilitation. RSD usually affects extremities and the return of function is as important as the short-term relief of symptoms and signs. The painful disabled limb should first be assessed to obtain a base-line. Such assessment is best carried out with the assistance of a trained therapist. Whenever possible, measurements should be made before and after all treatments to monitor the progress of the patient. If the therapist is present at each IVRG block, the patient can be encouraged to begin physical therapy from the moment the maximum response accrues.

REFERENCES

1. Hannington-Kiff, J.G. Intravenous regional sympathetic block with guanethidine. Lancet, 1: 1019-20, 1974.

2. Hannington-Kiff, J.G. Pain Relief. London: William Heinemann, 68-78, 1974.

3. Hannington-Kiff, J.G. Antisympathetic drugs in limbs. In: Wall P. D., Melzack R. eds., Textbook of Pain. Edinburgh: Churchill Livingstone, 566-73, 1984.

4. Hannington-Kiff, J.G. Prilocaine for Bier's block needs methylene-blue but not preservative. Lancet, 2: 1085, 1983.

5. Hannington-Kiff, J.G. Pharmacological target blocks in hand surgery and rehabilitation. Journal of Hand Surgery, 9-B: 29-36, 1984.

6. Hannington-Kiff, J.G. Pharmacological target blocks in painful dystrophic limbs. In: Wall P.D., Melzack R., eds., Textbook of Pain. 2nd Edition. Edinburgh: Churchill Livingstone, In Press.

7. Hannington-Kiff, J.G. In Limbo. Jacksonian Prize Dissertation 1980, *in libris* Royal College of Surgeons of England, London.

13

REFLEX SYMPATHETIC DYSTROPHY-NEUROSURGICAL APPROACHES

Ronald R. Tasker

This review will examine the surgical approaches to the treatment of neural injury pain especially as it relates to the sympathetic system. Difficulties arise when one attempts to fit RSD into this setting. RSD might be used to describe any complex of deafferentation or central pain, including posttraumatic syndrome where the neural injury element may be subclinical, which presents with sympathetic hyperfunction (1). RSD occurs in 5% of all cases of trauma (2). The term is often used interchangeably with Sudeck's atrophy (3), causalgia, minor causalgia, shoulder-hand syndrome, posttraumatic spreading neuralgia, posttraumatic pain, sympathalgia, chronic traumatic edema, algoneurodystrophy (1,4). It is precipitated by fracture in 50% of cases but blunt trauma, inflammation, laceration, surgery, soft tissue injury, injection, angina pectoris, vascular disease, myocardial infarct, osteoarthritis, frostbite and burns have all been identified causes. RSD may be diffuse or limited to a single finger; though commoner in adults, it also occurs in the young; it has been described in association with injuries to peripheral nerves, carpal and tarsal tunnel syndrome, lumbar and cervical disc disease, cord lesions, post-herpetic neuralgia and stroke (1,5-18). In a review of 333 consecutive personal cases of central and deafferentation pain (19), the author found evidence of sympathetic hyperfunction in 9 patients. It occurred in 1% of those with pain caused by nerve injury, 1% of the amputation-related group, and 1% of those with neural injury pain associated with disc disease. Two percent of patients with brachial plexus lesions and 4% of those with posttraumatic syndrome were affected. It was not seen in any of our patients with post-herpetic neuralgia, post-thoracotomy syndrome, peripheral vascular disease or central pain.

Invasive treatment of RSD usually consists of repeated sympathetic blocks and prognosis is generally considered better if the blocks can be done early in the course of the disease. Despite this, permanent sympathectomy is rarely successful in relieving pain (20-31).

Let us now look more closely at the curious group of pain syndromes included under the term neural injury pain: the deafferentation and central pains with which RSD may be associated. In some of these conditions, as Livingston (32) suggested, the neural injury element may be subclinical. This is the case in posttraumatic syndrome and incisional pain where, though small peripheral nerves are doubtless involved, neurological examination reveals no deficit. In other patients the neural element is much more obvious. Neural injury pain is idiosyncratic: that is, not all patients with a given neural lesion develop pain, and it is uncommon in the young. The onset of pain may be delayed after the causative event in 36 to 67% of patients with deafferentation pain, 77 to 86% with central pain. From 98 to 100% of patients suffer from a steady spontaneous pain that is usually burning and tingling in quality. Fourteen to 43% suffer from intermittent spontaneous pain whilst 19 to 88% suffer from evoked pain (hyperpathia, allodynia or hyperesthesia). These ranges reflect the different neural injury pain syndromes reviewed. The steady burning tingling element of RSD pain tends to be temporarily relieved by intravenous doses of sodium thiopental, insufficient to produce sleep. Though rarely relieved by opiates, the effect is not reversed by 0.4 to 0.8 mg of naloxone given intravenously. Proximal or distal local anesthetic somatosensory blockade usually relieves the pain temporarily, but it is important to recognise that permanent surgical denervation at the same site as the block, usually fails. Such burning tingling steady pain behaves as if it were caused by central neural aberrations such as denervation neuronal hypersensitivity caused in turn by the neural injury. Therapeutically it responds best to treatment with chronic stimulation. Curiously, only about 50% of apparently suitable candidates gain relief from chronic stimulation, indicating that there is a severe gap in our understanding of the pathophysiology. There is also <u>a tendency for patients to escape from control despite continued efficient operation of their stimulating device over time</u> so that the role of chronic stimulation appears to be to tide patients over a few years of extreme suffering until such time as their pain syndrome diminishes spontaneously.

Evoked pain behaves differently. Its nature is compatible with the normal stimulation of receptors but with aberrant central processing (34). It is relieved by neural interruption and possibly by opiates and spinothalamic section.

The intermittent pain behaves as if it were the result of ectopic impulses in afferent pathways arising at an injury site and appears to be relieved by afferent or spinothalamic interruption or else by opiates.

Surgical treatments of RSD presenting with causalgia as popularized by Leriche during World War I, have reportedly given relief varying from 22-97% (36). This experience led to the use of sympathectomy to treat other types of neural injury pain with or without sympathetic hyperfunction, which is usually unsuccessful (19,33). This despite the fact, that sympathetic blockade with either local anesthetic or guanethidine, temporarily relieves deafferentation and central pain in the presence of hyperpathia or allodynia (21,23,25), and for the concept of sympathetically maintained pain (36).

Major Causalgia

A rare entity in civilian practice, major causalgia was described by Weir Mitchell after the American Civil War (37) and has been thoroughly reviewed by Bonica (38). Major causalgia is usually the result of a partial lesion often caused by gunshot wound of the median or sciatic nerves or of the medial cord of the brachial plexus (37-41). The success rate of therapy with surgical sympathectomy varies from 12 to 97% in different series (1,4,23,39-43).

**Pain Caused by Peripheral Nerve Lesions
Other Than Major Causalgia**

These types of deafferentation pain are more common in civilian practice. Homans apparently introduced the term minor causalgia to describe those cases where accompanying sensory loss is complete (anesthesia dolorosa is another synonym often used). The term causalgic pain is often applied to this group of pains, causing both diagnostic confusion and use of inappropriate therapy. Though chronic stimulation of peripheral nerves, which requires open exposure of the nerve, is initially effective in 30 to 65% of cases, relief declines with time and is associated with the risk of various surgical complications (44-48).

Phantom and Stump Pain

The pain associated with amputation is difficult to treat (49-51). Sherman (52) reviewed a large series of U.S. servicemen with pain associated with amputation and found that sympathectomy yielded little enduring pain relief. After cordotomy 38% of patients were relieved and after thalamotomy 18%. Though Sherman's review and Iacono's experience (53) suggested that the DREZ procedure was useful in amputation-related pain, Saris et al. (54,55) pointed out clearly that results were good only if the amputation had been done for plexus avulsion. Fifty-six percent of this author's 16 patients with amputation pain, passed a trial of percutaneous cord stimulation and 56% went on to have enduring relief.

Post-herpetic Neuralgia

This distressing condition thoroughly reviewed by Loeser (56) responds poorly to denervation surgery (57).

Brachial Plexus Lesions

Though stretch and avulsion injuries are perhaps more familiar, lesions of any pathology can damage the brachial or lumbosacral plexus and cause deafferentation pain, with or without RSD. In stretch injuries, Wynn-Parry (59) found denervating surgery disappointing. Demierre and Siegfried (60) relieved 5 out of 7 patients suffering from pain caused by radiation necrosis of the brachial plexus with dorsal cord stimulation. In avulsion injuries but not in other types of lesion, Nashold and his group (58,61,62) have found 54% of 39 patients followed 1 to 8 years enjoying good sustained pain relief.

SUMMARY AND CONCLUSIONS

It is suggested that the term RSD be used to describe the 2% or so of patients with neural injury pain including posttraumatic syndrome associated with sympathetic hyperfunction. Except for major causalgia and the temporary relief of pain achieved by sympathetic block in some patients, surgical sympathectomy is not effective treatment for pain of reflex sympathetic dystrophy. In treating the accompanying pain, it is important to divide it into its component parts of steady, intermittent, shooting and evoked elements. Experience suggests that the steady burning tingling may have a central pathophysiology, say from denervation neuronal hypersensitivity, and be amenable to modulation with chronic stimulation. The intermittent shooting pain behaves as if due to ectopic impulses arising at an injury site, and the evoked pain to aberrant central processing of input through receptors. Both appear to respond to surgical interruption of sensory input, particularly spinothalamic input, and to the use of opiates or modulation of spinothalamic activity.

REFERENCES

1. Rowlingson, J.C. The sympathetic dystrophies. Int Anaesthesiol Clin, 321: 117-129, 1983.
2. Bonica, J.J. Causalgia and other reflex sympathetic dystrophies. In: Bonica, J.J., Liebeskind, J.C., Albe-Fessard, D.G. (eds.), Advances in Pain Research and Therapy, Vol. 3, New York, Raven, pp. 141-166, 1979.
3. Sudeck, P. Über die acute entzündliche Knoch enatrophie. Arch F Klin Chir, 62: 147-157, 1900.

4. Payne, R. Neuropathic pain syndromes, with special reference to causalgia and reflex sympathetic dystrophy. The Clin J of Pain, 2: 59-73, 1986.

5. Helms, C.A., O'Brien, E.T., Katzberg, R.W. Segmental reflex sympathetic dystrophy syndrome. Radiology, 135: 67-68, 1980.

6. Ruggeri, S.B., Athreya, B.H., Daughty, R., Gregg, J.R., Das, M.M. Reflex sympathetic dystrophy in children. Clin Orthopaedics and Related Research, 163: 225-230, 1982.

7. Buchta, R.M. Reflex sympathetic dystrophy in a 14-year-old female. J Adolescent Health Care, 4: 121-122, 1983.

8. Doolan, L.A., Brown, T.C.K. Reflex sympathetic dystrophy in a child. Anaesth Intens Care, 12: 70-72, 1984.

9. Chodoroff, B., Ball, R.D. Lumbosacral radiculopathy, reflex sympathetic dystrophy and tarsal tunnel syndrome; an unusual presentation. Arch Phys Med Rehab, 66: 185-187, 1985.

10. Dobritt, D.W., Hartrick, C.T. Reflex sympathetic dystrophy associated with multiple lumbar laminectomies. The Clin J of Pain, 2: 119-121, 1986.

11. Andrews, L.G., Armitage, K.J. Sudeck's atrophy in traumatic quadriplegia. Paraplegia, 9: 159-165, 1971-2.

12. Bentley, J.B., Hameroff, S.R. Diffuse reflex sympathetic dystrophy. Anesthesiology, 53: 256-257. 1980.

13. Swan, D.M. Shoulder-hand syndrome following hemiplegia. Neurology Minneap, 4: 480-482, 1954.

14. Ohry, A., Brooks, M.E., Steinbach, T.V., Rozin, R. Shoulder complications as a cause of delay in rehabilitation of spinal cord injured patients. Paraplegia, 16: 310-316, 1978-79.

15. Wainapel, S.F. Reflex sympathetic dystrophy following traumatic myelopathy. Pain, 18: 345-349, 1984.

16. Van Ouwenaller, C., Laplace, P.M., Chantraine A. Painful shoulder in hemiplegia. Arch Phys Med Rehab, 67: 23-26, 1967.

17. Grossleght, K.R., Rowlingson, J.C., Boaden, R.W. Herpes zoster and reflex sympathetic dystrophy. Anesth Analg, 65: 309-311, 1986.

18. Moskowitz, E., Bishop, H.F., Pe, H., Shibutani, K. Posthemiplegic reflex sympathetic dystrophy. JAMA, June 14: 836-839, 1958.

19. Tasker, R.R., Dostrovsky, J.O. Deafferentation and central pain. In: Wall, P.D., Melzack, R. (eds.), Textbook of pain, 2nd ed. Churchill Livingstone, Edinburgh. (in press)

20. Hannington-Kiff, J. Intravenous regional sympathetic block with guanethidine. Lancet, 1: 1019-1020, 1974.

21. Nathan, P.W. Improvement in cutaneous sensitivity associated with relief of pain. J Neurol Neurosurg Psychiat, 23: 202-206, 1960.

22. Bergan, J.J., Conn, J.J.R. Sympathectomy for pain relief. Medical Clinics of North America, 52: 145-159, 1968.

23. Loh, L., Nathan, P.W., Schott, G.D. Pain due to lesions of central nervous system removed by sympathetic block. Brit Med J, 282: 1026-1028, 1981.

24. Glynn, C.J., Basedow, R.W., Walsh, J.A. Pain relief following post-ganglionic sympathetic blockage with IV guanethidine. Brit J Anaesth, 53: 1297-1302, 1981.

25. Loh, L., Nathan, P.W. Painful peripheral states and sympathetic blocks. J Neurol Neurosurg Psychiat, 41: 661-671, 1978.

26. Subbarao, J., Stillwell, G.K. Reflex sympathetic dystrophy syndrome of the upper extremity: Analysis of total outcome of management of 125 cases. Arch Phys Med Rehab, 62: 549-554, 1981.

27. Driessen, J.J., van der Werken, C., Nicolai, J.P.A., Crul, J.F. Clinical effects of regional intravenous guanethidine (ismelin R) in reflex sympathetic dystrophy. Acta Anaesthesiol Scan, 27: 505-509, 1983.

28. Ficat, P., Nedjar, C., Sarre, J., Villa, P.L. Le traitement de l'algodystrophie reflexe par bloc intraveineux. Chir Orthop, 69: 83-88, 1983.

29. Linson, M.A., Leffert, R., Todd, D.P. The treatment of upper extremity reflex sympathetic dystrophy with prolonged continuous stellate ganglion blockade. The J of Hand Surgery, 8: 153-159, 1983.

30. Schutzer, S.F., Gossling, H.R. The treatment of reflex sympathetic dystrophy syndrome. J of Bone and Joint Surgery, 66A: 625-629, 1984.

31. Wang, J.K., Johnson, K.A., Itstrup, D.M. Sympathetic blocks for reflex sympathetic dystrophy. Pain, 23: 13-17, 1985.

32. Livingston, W.K. Pain mechanisms: A physiological interpretation of causalgia and its related states. Macmillan, New York, 1943.

33. Tasker, R. R. Management of nociceptive, deafferentation and central pain by surgical intervention. In: Fields, H. (ed.), Pain Syndromes in Neurological Practice. Butterworths, London. (in press)

34. Lindblom, U. Assessment of abnormal evoked pain in neurological pain patients and its relation to spontaneous pain: A descriptive and conceptual model with some analytical results. In: Fields, H.L., Dubner, R., Cervero, R. (eds.), Advances in Pain Research and Therapy, Vol. 9, pp. 402-423, 1985.

35. Sweet, W.H. Causalgia: Sympathetic dystrophy (Sudeck's atrophy). In: Wilkins, R.H., Rengachary, S.S (eds.). Neurosurgery. McGraw-Hill, New York, pp. 1886-1893, 1985.

36. Roberts, W.J. A hypothesis on the physiological basis for causalgia and related pains. Pain, 24, 297-311, 1986.

37. Weir, M.S. Injuries of nerves and their consequences. Dover, New York. Reproduction of the first edition by J. B. Lippincott and Co., Philadelphia, 1965.

38. Bonica, J.J. Causalgia and other reflex sympathetic dystrophies. In: Bonica, J.J., Liebeskind, J.C., Albe-Fessard, D.G. (eds.), Advances in Pain Research and Therapy, Vol. 3, Raven, New York, 141-166, 1979.

39. Nathan, P.W. On the pathogenesis of causalgia in peripheral nerve lesions. Brain, 70: 145-170, 1947.

40. Noordenbos, W. Pain, Elsevier, Amsterdam, 1959.

41. Sunderland, S. Pain mechanisms in causalgia. J Neurol Neurosurg Psychiat, 39: 471-480, 1976.

42. Shumaker, H.B., Jr. A personal view of causalgia and other reflex dystrophies. Ann Surg, 201: 278-289, 1985.

43. Tahmoush, A.J. Causalgia: Redefinition as a clinical pain syndrome. Pain, 10: 187-197, 1981.

44. Campbell, J.N., Long, D.M. Peripheral nerve stimulation in the treatment of intractable pain. J Neurosurg, 45: 692-699, 1946.

45. Picaza, J.A. Peripheral nerve stimulation for pain control. J Florida Medical Ass, 63: 903-905, 1976.

46. Picaza, J.A., Cannon, B.W., Hunter, S.E., Boyd, A.S, Gunna, J., Maurer, D. Pain suppression by peripheral nerve stimulation, Part III: Observations with implanted devices. Surgical Neurology, 4: 115-126, 1975.

47. Picaza, J.A., Hunter, J.E., Cannon, B.W. Session in peripheral nerve and neuromuscular stimulation. Pain suppression: Chronic effects. Neurology, 1: 226-227, 1977.

48. Picaza, J.A., Hunter, S.E., Cannon, B.W. Pain suppression by peripheral nerve stimulation. Chronic effects of implanted devices. Appl Neurophysiol, 40: 223-234, 1977-8.

49. Carlen, P.L., Wall, P.D., Nodvorna, H., Steinbach, T. Phantom limbs and related phenomena in recent traumatic amputations. Neurol Minneap, 28: 211-217, 1978.

50. Siegfried, J., Cetinalp, E. Neurosurgical treatment of phantom limb pain: A survey of methods. In: Siegfried, J., Zimmermann, M. (eds.). Phantom and Stump Pain. Springer Verlag, Berlin, pp. 148-155, 1981.

51. Jansen, T.S, Rasmussen, P. Amputation. In: Wall, P.D., Melzack, R. (eds.), Textbook of Pain. Churchill Livingstone, Edinburgh, pp. 402-412, 1984.

52. Sherman, R.A., Sherman, C.J., Parker, L. Chronic phantom and stump pain among American veterans: Results of a survey. Pain, 18: 83-95, 1984.

53. Iacono, R.P., Linford, J., Sandyk, R. Pain management after lower extremity amputation. Neurosurgery, 20: 496-500, 1987.

54. Saris, S.C., Iacono, R.P., Nashold, B.S., Jr. Dorsal root entry zone lesions for post amputation pain. J Neurosurg, 62: 72-76, 1985.

55. Saris, S.C., Iacono, R.P., Nashold, B.S., Jr. Successful treatment of phantom pain with dorsal root entry zone coagulation. Appl Neurophysiol, 51: 1188-1197, 1988.

56. Loeser, J.D. Herpes zoster and postherpetic neuralgia. Pain, 25: 149-164, 1986.

57. Demierre, B., Siegfried, J. Traitement neurochirurgical de la neuralgie postherpetiforme. Médécine et Hygiene, 41: 1960-1965, 1983.

58. Nashold, B.S., Jr., Ostdahl, R.H., Bullitt, E., Friedman, A., Brophy, B. Dorsal root entry zone lesions: A new neurosurgical therapy for deafferentation pain. In: Bonica, J.J., Lindblom, U., Iggo, A. (eds.), Advances in Pain Research and Therapy, Vol. 5, Raven, New York, pp. 739-750, 1983.

59. Wynn-Parry, C.B. Management of pain in avulsion lesions of the brachial plexus. In: Bonica, J.J., Lindblom, U., Iggo, A. (eds.), Advances in Pain Research and Therapy, Vol. 5, Raven, New York, pp. 751-761, 1983.

60. Demierre, B., Siegfried, J. Douleurs après irradiation therapeutique. Discussion des mecanismes et proposition de traitement. Medecine et Hygiene, 42: 1777-1782, 1984.

61. Nashold, B.S., Jr., Ostdahl, R.H. Dorsal root entry zone lesions for pain relief. J Neurosurg, 51: 59-69, 1979.

62. Friedman, A.H., Bullitt, E. Dorsal root entry zone lesions in the treatment of pain following brachial plexus avulsion, spinal cord injury and herpes zoster. Appl Neurophysiol, 51: 164-169, 1988.

14

PERIPHERAL NERVE STIMULATOR IMPLANT FOR TREATMENT OF RSD

Gabor B. Racz, Boyce Lewis, Jr.,
James E. Heavner and John Scott

Injury to peripheral nerves may produce causalgia as described in detail in preceding chapters. Sweet and Wepsic (1,2) utilized electrical stimulation to treat causalgia involving the median and ulnar nerves, to produce a pleasant "tingling" and loss of the burning pain in many cases.

Subsequently, surgical techniques were developed for implanting two different types of peripheral nerve stimulating electrodes for treating causalgia (3,4). Varying success rates were reported with these electrodes; for instance, 58% (5) and 52.6% for upper extremity and 31% pain relief for lower extremity pain (4,6). However, foreign body reactions related to direct electrode contact with the nerve, was one limitation to the usefulness of this therapy. A surgical implantation technique was therefore developed, that creates a barrier between the nerve and the electrode, by covering the electrode with a thin fibrous membrane from intramuscular septa. The stimulator also has the capacity to be periodically cycled and to change pulse width.

In this chapter, the surgical technique is described, together with observations from neuro-physiological recordings made via the implanted electrode during the initial trial stimulation phase.

Patient Selection and Electrode Placement

Patients assessed as having reflex sympathetic dystrophy, and seen in consultation with orthopedic surgery, proceeded to a surgical stimulator implant, carried out under general anesthesia. The first stage was placement of the Resume lead under the affected nerve proximal to the site of injury. Electrodes were placed at either the median or ulnar nerves-4-5 cm proximal to the medial epicondyle; saphenous nerve--approximately 15 cm proximal to the knee; and tibialis nerve 3-4 cm above the ankle. A section of the nerve approximately 4 cm long is dissected free and a flap created from adjacent fascia, usually from the intramuscular septum, which is folded over the electrode to prevent direct contact between the electrode and the nerve. The electrode is placed directly underneath the nerve and is separated from it by the fascia. The nerve is allowed to return to its normal position in such a way that it lies directly over the electrode. Several soft tissue elements are then sutured loosely over the nerve to maintain close contact between the nerve and the electrode. The electrode lead is externalized and connected to a temporary electrical stimulator (standard screener model #3623, Medtronic).

Electrode Stimulation Requirements

When the patient awakens from anesthesia, temporary stimulation is begun; the pattern, voltage, duration and contact points, through which stimulation is applied, are varied as necessary to obtain the desired response.

Temporary stimulation is evaluated for three days. Pain relief, mobilization and restoration of sleep patterns are early measures of response. If the patient and physicians are satisfied with the response, a permanent Itrel (Medtronic) programmable stimulating battery pack is implanted under general anesthesia as a second procedure.

Battery Pack Implantation

The battery pack is implanted near to the site of stimulation, either in the upper chest wall, the lower quadrant of the abdomen, or in the thigh approximately over Hunter's canal, depending on which nerve is being stimulated. Initial settings of the Itrel unit are as follows: amplitude, 0.75 to 1.25 volt; pulse width, 190 to 400 microseconds; pulse rate, 65 to 85 pulses per second; cycling, time on-64 seconds and time off-2 minutes, soft-start on. The appropriate amplitude is found by increasing the stimulus intensity by 0.25 volt increments until the patient reports a perception of stimulation. Optimal settings are further fine-tuned by increasing or decreasing the pulse width.

Patients and Preliminary Results

Twenty-four implants have been placed in 23 patients (11 female, 12) male). The follow-up period to date ranges from 1 to 15 months. For the most part, their nerve injuries were either work, accident or sports related, though a iatrogenic component was noted in some. Time from injury to implant ranged from 5 months to 10 years. A total of 14 pain-related surgeries on the females and 23 surgeries on the males were previously undertaken. None of the surgeries had provided lasting benefit.

The patient's rating of pain intensity on a linear analog scale (0-10) was reduced significantly following the initiation of stimulation in most patients regardless of sex, duration of pain or cause. Hyper-sensitivity, back spasms and functional limitation were reduced in one female but her pain scores did not change because all four extremities were painful. The male who benefited least from the implant most likely had pain of iatrogenic origin and was involved in an associated lawsuit. Opioid use was also significantly reduced in all cases. Two of the 11 females have returned to work, as have six of the 12 males. We expect more of the patients to return to work on completion of their physical therapy. Two of the 23 patients have required reoperation, one for a broken wire, the other for a leak in the insulation.

Recording From Implanted Electrode

Background. Direct recordings from nerves supplying areas where patients have persistent pain may contribute to our understanding of why the pain persists. Recordings from neurons in animals have revealed that C-fibers in damaged nerves have spontaneous activity and generate mechanosensitive ectopic discharges (7). Microneurographic techniques have been used in humans to limited extent to study neural activity in pain patients (8). Such recordings in a patient with causalgia revealed neither an abnormal increase nor abnormal pattern of sympathetic outflow to the hyperalgetic skin (9).

Recording Technique. Recordings were made as follows:

a) Supine and resting (spontaneous activity).

b) Movement of the affected extremity (movement).

c) Tactile stimulation in the area supplied by the nerve (cutaneous stimulation response).

With patient consent, we record as many as three sessions from each patient, starting immediately after electrode implantation or on the first postoperative day. Recording sessions are done at 24-hour intervals.

Results. Recordings have been made from nine patients ages 24 to 69 years old, six males and three females, all caucasian. In four cases, recordings were made from the tibial nerve, two from the ulnar nerve, and three from the median. The electrode was implanted proximal to the initial injury site in six instances and very near to or distal to the initial injury site in three instances.

All patients reported that aside from pain at the electrode implantation site, they were pain-free within 24 hours of starting continuous stimulation. Pain usually returned within a few minutes after the stimulation was stopped for the recording sessions. However, the pain-free period increased with successive recording sessions.

Four prominent types of spontaneous recordings were obtained: 1) none (N = 2); 2) sharp waveforms rising from a nearly flat baseline occurring at a relatively fixed interval (N = 2); 3) rounded waveforms occurring continuously (N = 2); randomly but frequently occurring sharp waveforms (N = 3). Movement of an appendage in the pain site generally increased the amplitude and/or frequency of the signal. In one case where there was no spontaneous activity, movement produced spike-like activity. Tactile exploration of the cutaneous area innervated by the nerve with the electrode implant elicited a clear-cut response in only a few patients. In one case there was evidence that the medial nerve cutaneous receptive field had expanded into radial and ulnar nerve areas.

We tentatively conclude from the recordings that spontaneous nerve activity in patients relates to the pain syndrome. One patient (pain duration 10 years) from whom no spontaneous activity was recorded, reflexly extended the contralateral leg when the tibial nerve was stimulated. Also electrical stimulation of the nerve elicited after-discharge activity in muscle recordings from this patient. These findings suggest that changes had occurred within the central nervous system and that peripheral nerve function was normal. The other patient (pain duration six months) in whom no spontaneous activity was recorded, had no obvious physical damage associated with the initial event that triggered the pain syndrome. The recordings offer no explanation for this patient's pain.

These limited observations are consistent with suggestions that spontaneous nerve activity may be associated with certain pain states and may be casually related to the nociception (afferent) or its sequelae (efferent; swelling, edema, vasoconstriction). In those patients, peripheral nerve stimulation may provide pain relief by blocking the spontaneous nerve activity (collision) and/or via spinal cord mechanisms (e.g., "spinal gate"). It is important to keep in mind that stimulation intensity used for peripheral nerve stimulation is usually set at threshold for sensation, i.e., only activates large myelinated fibers not normally associated with pain perception. Therefore, a suggestion that collision is a mechanism for pain relief implies a belief that the pain syndrome is mediated, at least in part, via the large nerve fibers.

DISCUSSION

We believe the method of peripheral nerve stimulation described in this chapter represents an improvement on the original technique described by Sweet and Wepsic in 1967. Technological advances as described, and the better batteries, are now able to maintain continuous programmable stimulation for several years. This surgical approach to the electrode implantation, is felt to not only avoid scar formation, but also to induce changes in the nervous system which might lead to sustained pain relief.

The patients included in this series all had experience with transcutaneous electrical stimulation (TENS) prior to referral to our clinic. None of them benefited from this therapy. There would therefore appear to be little correlation between the results of TENS and peripheral nerve stimulator implants (10).

Recordings made from the implanted electrodes suggest that changes occur in peripheral nerves and in the central nervous system, in patients with causalgia. The presence of spontaneous activity in the peripheral nerve when the patient is inactive could lead one to believe that the sympathetic response is a consequence of activity generated by the injured nerve (terminal or axon). Indeed, it is possible to see a very rapid reversal of the hyperhidrosis, vasoconstriction and allodynia, as soon as peripheral nerve stimulation is started. The spontaneous discharge of axons may be inhibited by stimulation of the nerve at the appropriate location or the consequence of the spontaneous firing may be negated at the spinal cord level by the appropriate stimulation.

* Note. Discussion recognised the limited follow-up of these patients and readers are referred to Tasker's review of this topic and its less than encouraging outlook in previous reported studies. (Chapter 13) Eds.

REFERENCES

1. Sweet, W.H., Wepsic, J.B. Trans Am Neurol Assoc, 93: 103, 1968.
2. White, J.C., Sweet, W.H. Pain and the Neurosurgeon: A forty year experience. Charles C. Thomas, Springfield, IL, pp. 895-896, 1969.
3. Picaza, J. A., et al. Surg Neurol, 4: 115-126, 1975.
4. Nashold, B.S., Goldner, J.L., Mullen, J.B., Bright, D.S. J Bone Joint Surg, 64-A: 1-10, 1985.
5. Waisbrod, H., Panhans, C.H., Hansen, D., Gerbershagen, H.U. J Bone Joint Surg, 67-B: 470-472, 1985.

6. Hunt, J.L. In: Salisbury, R.E. (ed.), Burns of the Upper Extremity, W. B. Saunders, Philadelphia, pp. 72-83, 1976.

7. Blumberg, H., Jänig, W. Pain, 20: 335-353, 1984.

8. Torebjörk, E.K., Hallin, R.G. In: Bonica, J.J. et al. (eds.), Advances in Pain Research and Therapy, Raven Press, New York, pp. 121-131, 1979.

9. Wallin, G., Torebjörk, H.E., Hallen, R.G. In: Zotterman, Y. (ed.), Sensory Function of the Skin in Primates with Special Reference to Man. Pergamon Press, Oxford, pp. 489-502, 1976.

10. Fields, H.L. Pain. McGraw-Hill Book Company, New York, p. 319, 1987.

15

PSYCHOLOGIC SUPPORT OF THE PATIENT
WITH REFLEX SYMPATHETIC DYSTROPHY

J. David Haddox

As has already been stated in Chapters 2 and 5, the psychological aspects of reflex sympathetic dystrophy have not been systematically studied in sufficient detail to provide an accurate and reliable portrayal of the disease from a behavioral medicine standpoint. Most of the literature that addresses this aspect is anecdotal in nature. Few studies have been done using psychometric instruments, and they have failed to differentiate these patients from patients suffering with chronic pain of other etiologies (1).

In reviewing the studies in which the emotional aspects of RSD have been noted, one is impressed by the number of reports from non-psychiatrists that comment on psychologic issues. Poplawski, et al. studied sixty-two patients and stated that all of them showed some degree of anxiety (2). Schwartzman and McLellan comment in a recent review article on the anxious nature of patients with RSD (3). Several other authors have made similar observations (4-7). Holden felt that patients suffering from RSD are "discouraged and apprehensive" (8), while Clark advocated treating depression as a major part of the overall approach (9). Spero and Schwartz have also noted these patients to be depressed (5).

The sense of hopelessness experienced by these patients bears mention as well. Shumacker and Abramson remarked on the "relatively hopeless viewpoint" that was held by the majority of their 142 patients with RSD (12). They theorized that this feeling of hopelessness stemmed from long-term disability, with a concomitant dim view of eventual recovery--a condition they referred to as "chronic invalidism." The Reflex Sympathetic Dystrophy Syndrome Association, in their brochure "RSDS - The Pain That Doesn't Stop," lists as effects of RSD, frustration, anger, exhaustion, and hopelessness for the patient and the family.

PSYCHOTHERAPY

The need for psychotherapy to be administered con current with somatic interventions, such as sympathetic blockade, has been addressed by Omer (10), Rizzi, et al. (11) and Clark (9). The opinion of these writers was that the psychologic distress of RSD was sufficient to warrant direct treatment, coincident with therapy aimed at the sympathetic nervous system per se.

Supportive Therapy

Supportive therapy can and should be provided to patients and families not only by psychologists and psychiatrists, but by all staff who work in the pain clinic setting. In order to do this effectively, the belief systems of the staff members must be in concert with what is currently known about the psychologic aspects of medical diseases. Too often, a response to psychologic intervention is misconstrued to be prima facie evidence of a psychiatric problem. This may then result in the patient being treated in a different manner than if he or she had a "real" (organic) disease. This hearkens to the Cartesian concept of the mind-body dichotomy which is not valid today. It is well known that behavioral or psychologic issues and treatments can influence the course of medical diseases (13,14). Lehman, in report of four cases of RSD in 1934, stated aptly: "There is, of course, a psychic element in every injury and disease" (15). It is up to the treatment team to embrace this notion and to accept the psyche as part of the patient.

Due to the disparity between patient complaints and the expected clinical course of the inciting event, (fracture, sprain, carpal tunnel release, etc.) the patient often receives messages that the pain is psychogenic (2,3,5,16-20).

Occasionally, the implication is that the patient with RSD is even a malingerer (20,21). By knowing that the patient and family have likely been exposed to this, staff can reduce a great amount of hostility and anxiety, by stated recognition that their pain is "real" and not some imaginary fabrication.

Stress Reduction

Another area of supportive therapy that the staff can utilize is that of overall stress reduction. It is known that indicators of stress correlate with utilization of health care services (22). It is also presumed that emotional stress causes sympathetic nervous system activity to increase to the point where it could have an adverse effect on the peripheral manifestations of RSD (2,3,5,8,12,18,19,23). Interviewing the patient with this in mind can help the staff identify and reduce or eliminate sources of stress in the clinic setting. The psychotherapist can help the patient examine his or her life for sources of stress and reaction patterns to that stress. Stress, of course, can never be totally eliminated from a person's life, but the way in which a person responds can be altered with any of several stress management protocols.

SOCIAL SUPPORT SYSTEMS

Social support systems should be identified and strengthened where possible. The usual sources of this support are family and friends, but other avenues of social support may be available. The clinic staff will, in many cases, function as another realm of support for the patient with RSD that has been refractory to somatic therapies. Individual relationships with members of the treatment team can be quite useful in helping the patient cope with his situation. Groups for pain patient support can be provided on an outpatient basis, and may provide a first step for reentry into social spheres for the RSD patient, who some authors have described as being socially withdrawn (3). The importance of social support systems should not be underestimated. In a recent study of visit patterns in a health maintenance organization, social support was shown to be correlated with a decreased number of visits in a high stress cohort of adults, as compared to a similar stress level group with less perceived social support (22). This data supports a construct that is evolving in the behavioral medicine literature, that is that social support buffers against the adverse effects of stress on health. Pursuant to pain patients, a study of coping styles in tension headache sufferers compared to controls found that the headache patients used more passive mechanisms for coping with interpersonal stress, such as not seeking social support (24).

Staff Support

An area of supportive therapy of the patient with RSD that deserves comment is that of intra-staff support. As health care providers, we often pride ourselves on our ability to diagnose and treat diseases to provide favorable outcomes. This is especially true of pain clinicians, who regularly deal with conditions that are obscure to much of the rest of medicine. When con fronted with a patient who has a long-standing RSD, we must be cognizant of our own feelings and how this may affect our interactions with our patient. At the outset, there may be feelings of anger that the patient wasn't referred earlier when sympathetic blocks would have had a better chance of success. Expressing this anger and frustration directly or indirectly to the patient will serve to reinforce his belief that he has been mismanaged, and is still suffering through someone else's negligence. A second issue in this regard is that these patients may not get better, despite our ministrations. This challenges the professional ego, and, if not recognized and dealt with effectively, can lead to poor therapeutic decisions and staff "burn-out".

SELF CONCEPT

Bandura has popularized the concept of self-efficacy expectancy (25). This is defined as the degree of conviction an individual has in his/her ability to successfully complete a given task. A high self-efficacy expectancy is thought to correlate with increased pain tolerance (26,27). Social modeling can lead to improved self-efficacy expectancy (28). This can enhance the patient's confidence that he or she will be able to handle a flare-up of their pain, complete a chore, etc, and will contribute to improved self-esteem. 29).

SUMMARY

In summary, it can be said that supportive psycho therapy has a place in the management of RSD. Careful studies are needed to delineate how much this can contribute to the treatment of these patients. In such studies, it is critical that reasonable outcome measures be employed, since simplistic variables (e.g., visual analog scale scores) may be misleading when examining the more chronic forms of RSD.

"Above all it must be recognized that the patient with RSD (causalgia) depends on a definable person for help, and they respond favorably to such interest, whether it be from a physician, therapist or social worker. If this lifeline of care is broken, there will be very little hope for recovery, and hope is what all patients need most" (9).

REFERENCES

1. Haddox, J.D. (in press). Psychological aspects of reflex sympathetic dystrophy. In Stanton-Hicks, M.D. (ed.), Reflex sympathetic dystrophy. Boston: Kluwer Academic Publishers.

2. Poplawski, Z.J., Wiley, A.M., Murray, J.F. Post-Traumatic dystrophy of the extremities: A clinical review and trial of treatment." J. Bone Jt. Surg. 65-A: 642-655, 1983.

3. Schwartzman, R.J., McLellan, T. L. Reflex sympathetic dystrophy: A review. Arch. Neurol. 44: 555-561, 1987.

4. Pak, T.J., Martin, G.M., Magness, J.L., Kavanaugh, G.J. Reflex sympathetic dystrophy: Review of 140 cases. Minn. Med. 53: 507-512, 1970.

5. Spero, M.W., Schwartz, E. Psychiatric aspects of foot problems. In Jahss, M.H. (ed.), Disorders of the foot. Philadelphia: Saunders, 1982.

6. Erickson, J.C. Evaluation and management of autonomic dystrophies of the upper extremity. In Hunter, J.M., Schneider, L.H., Macklin, E.J., Bell, J.A. (eds.), Rehabilitation of the hand. St. Louis: Mosby, 1978.

7. Steinbrocker, O., Argyros, T.G. The shoulder-hand syndrome: Present status as a diagnostic and therapeutic entity. Med. Clin. N. Am., 4: 1533-1553, 1958.

8. Holden, W.D. Sympathetic dystrophy. Arch. Surg. 57: 373-384, 1948.

9. Clark, G.L. Causalgia: A discussion of the chronic pain syndromes in the upper limb. In Hunter, J.M., Schneider, L.H., Macklin, E.J., Bell, J.A. (eds.), Rehabilitation of the hand. St. Louis: Mosby, 1978.

10. Omer, G.E. Management of pain syndromes in the upper extremity. In Hunter, J.M., Schneider, L.H., Macklin, E.J., Bell, J.A. (eds.), Rehabilitation of the hand. St. Louis: Mosby, 1978.

11. Rizzi, R. Visentin, M., Mazzetti, G. Reflex sympathetic dystrophy. In Benedetti, C., Chapman, C.R., Moricca, G. (eds.) Advances in Pain Research and Therapy, Vol. 7. New York: Raven Press, 1984.

12. Shumacker, H.B., Abramson, D.I. Posttraumatic vasomotor disorders. Surg. Gyn. Ob. 88: 417-434, 1949.

13. Glaser, R., Kiecolt-Glaser, J.K., Speicher, C.E., Holliday, J.E. Stress, loneliness, and changes in herpesvirus latency. J. Behav. Med. 8 (3): 249-260, 1985.

14. Blanchard, E.B., McCoy, G.C., Wittrock, D., Musso, A., Gerardi, R.J., Pangburn, L. A controlled comparison of thermal biofeedback and relaxation training in the treatment of essential hypertension: II. Effects on cardiovascular reactivity. Health Psychol. 7 (1): 19-33, 1988.

15. Lehman, E.P. Traumatic vasospasm: A study of four cases of vasospasm in the upper extremity. Arch. Surg. 29: 92-107, 1934.

16. Wirth, F.P., Rutherford, R.B. A civilian experience with causalgia. Arch. Surg. 100 (6): 633-638, 1970.

17. Grunert, B.K., Devine, C.A., Sanger, J.R., Matloub, H.S., Green, D. Thermal self-regulation for pain control in reflex sympathetic dystrophy syndrome. Read at Eighteenth Annual Meeting of American Association for Hand Surgery, Toronto, 1988.

18. Bonica, J.J. Causalgia and other reflex sympathetic dystrophies. In Bonica, J.J., Liebeskind, J.C., Albe-Fessard, D.G. (eds.), Advances in pain research and therapy, Vol. 3. New York: Raven Press, 1979.

19. Miller, D.S., de Takats, G. Posttraumatic dystrophy of the extremities: Sudeck's atrophy. Surg. Gyn. Ob. 75: 558-582, 1942.

20. Uematsu, S., Hendler, N., Hungerford, D., Long, D., Ono, N. Thermography and electromyography in the differential diagnosis of chronic pain syndromes and reflex sympathetic dystrophy. Electromyogr. Clin. Neurophysiol. 21: 165-182, 1981.

21. Lankford, L.L. Reflex sympathetic dystrophy of the upper extremity. In Flynn, J.E. (ed.), Hand surgery, 3rd Ed. Baltimore: Williams and Wilkins, 1982.

22. Pilisuk, M., Boylan, R., Acredolo, C. Social support, life stress, and subsequent medical care utilization. Health Psychol. 6 (4): 273-288, 1987.

23. Doupe, J., Cullen, C.H., Chance, G.Q. Post- traumatic pain and the causalgic syndrome. J. Neurol. Neurosurg. Psychiat. 7: 33-48, 1944.

24. Murphy, A.I., Lehrer, P.M. Coping styles of muscle-contraction headache sufferers: Cognitive and physiological mechanisms. Read at Ninety-Fourth Annual Convention of American Psychological Association, Washington.

25. Bandura, A. Self-efficacy mechanism in human agency. Am. Psychol. 37: 122-147, 1977.

26. Taylor, M.L. Self-efficacy training in a multidisciplinary setting. Read at the Twelfth Scientific Meeting of the Midwest Pain Society, Milwaukee, 1981.

27. Litt, M.D. Self-efficacy and perceived control: Cognitive mediators of pain tolerance. Read at the Society of Behavioral Medicine, Washington, 1987.

28. Craig, K.D. Social modeling influences: Pain in context. In Sternbach, R.A. (ed.), The psychology of pain, 2nd ed. New York: Raven Press, 1986.

29. Haddox, J.D. The problems in overlapping professional roles in pain management. Read at the Tenth Scientific Meeting of the Midwest Pain Society, Las Vegas, 1986.

16

REFLEX SYMPATHETIC DYSTROPHY
NON-INVASIVE METHODS OF TREATMENT

J. E. Charlton

Introduction

There are many non-invasive treatment modalities suggested for the management of reflex sympathetic dystrophy [RSD]. It is unusual for a single treatment to be offered, and polytherapy is the rule rather than the exception. This suggests that no single treatment is likely to be effective, and that the cause and presentation are multifactorial.

The precipitating causes of RSD are protean and have been extensively reviewed (1-4). Virtually every paper published on the topic emphasises the importance of early recognition and restoration of normal function as the key to successful management. It is recommended usually that this be achieved by a combination of sympathetic blockade and vigorous physiotherapy.

Treatment of the Precipitating Injury

It is axiomatic that treatment of the local injury takes precedence over active physiotherapy. This includes treatment at the site of the injury and the relief of acute pain. Proper care of the local injury may require debridement, removal of foreign bodies, adequate reduction and decompression of fractures, surgical correction of torn muscles, tendons and ligaments, early repair of the neural injury and active treatment of any infection. The use of regional anaesthetic techniques may be particularly appropriate in this context as it may lead to less postoperative pain (5). It is interesting to speculate whether the increased use of regional techniques for trauma surgery would lead to fewer chronic painful sequelae as has been described for phantom limb pain (6,7).

Physiotherapy

There is widespread agreement that physiotherapy is a vital part of any treatment programme. A wide variety of treatment methods have been used but there are no adequate comparative studies and it is rare for this treatment to be used alone. Frequently "physiotherapy" is used as a generic term and one is left with the impression that no clear instructions accompany the patient to the physiotherapy department. It is rare for there to be mention of assessment, comparison of treatments, control groups or a rational to the choice of one treatment or another. Documentation of the use of physiotherapy is a matter of anecdotal reminiscence and unsupported prejudice.

There are reports that suggest that physiotherapy alone can be sufficient therapy for mild cases of RSD. Baker and Winegarner reported the successful treatment of 6 of 28 patients with physiotherapy (8). They emphasised that early institution of treatment gave a greater chance of success, and they felt the physiotherapist should be both aggressive and enthusiastic. The reviews of Omer and Thomas (9) and Pak et al. (10) also report successful resolution of RSD with physiotherapy alone in some cases. However, the nature of the successful physiotherapy varied and included elevation, traction, individual splints, exercising devices and something termed "general body conditioning."

Lindblom has pointed out (11) that the hyperalgesia found in RSD is not confined to mechanical stimuli. Thus, it is not surprising that both cold and heat have been advocated as treatment.

Cold

Cold wet compresses are mentioned in Mitchell's original article (12). The "wet towel sign" is a well known presentation in which the patient wraps his or her affected extremity in a cold damp towel to try and obtain some symptomatic relief from the constant burning pain. Ice packs were part of the treatment regimen described by Chan and Chow in their study of electroacupuncture in the treatment of RSD (13).

This study serves as an example of the problems which may be encountered in assessing the use of non-invasive therapy. Prior to their participation in the trial of electroacupuncture the twenty study patients were described as having at least one month of treatment with unspecified analgesics and intensive physiotherapy (active exercise, gentle passive mobilisation, massage and ice-packs). Careful assessment of function was carried out during the trial of electroacupuncture, but there is nothing to suggest that this was carried out before any of the other treatment employed.

Rather than being of benefit, it is more likely that hyperalgesia to cooling stimuli may characterise patients with sympathetic dystrophy, as demonstrated in an elegant study by Frost and her co-workers (14). These workers believe that patients with pain from mild cooling stimuli are likely to have a sympathetically-maintained component to their pain and may benefit from procedures directed at reducing sympathetic input into the painful area.

Heat

Heat is a common part of physiotherapy and is applied in the form of local or distant heat. Local heat by radiant lamps, heated water baths, paraffin or wax baths may produce a large number of local responses, many of which may be induced by changes in blood flow. There may be additional advantages to such therapy, such as the buoyancy of the water in a whirlpool bath permitting more exercise of painful joints. Distant heating can be achieved by ultrasound, interferential or short-wave diathermy. Care must be taken with the use of heat as there is potential for tissue damage. The topic of using heat and cold for therapeutic purposes has been reviewed recently by Lehman (15).

The usual goal of therapy is to improve function and increase the range of movements in the painful area. Inevitably, this means that both passive and active assisted exercises are employed in combination with superficial heat, ultrasound and other therapy such as drugs and sympathetic blocks (16-20).

The use of physiotherapy is non-specific, and usually, is not carried out under the direct supervision of the referring physician.

Immobilisation

By contrast, the decision to immobilise a limb with RSD is an active one on the part of the physician. With one exception (21), immobilisation has never been shown to have any beneficial effect upon the disease process and in many cases made matters worse (17,18,22-25). This finding agrees with the suggestion that it is possible to provoke physical findings very similar to RSD by totally immobilising a healthy limb for a prolonged period (Butler, S.H., personal communication.

The beneficial role of physiotherapy is virtually indisputable, and if there is any total agreement in the literature it is that active physiotherapy should not be taken to excess as this carries the risk of making matters worse. Thus, adequate analgesia is a prerequisite for successful physiotherapy. Whether it is the physiotherapy, or the analgesia that permits the physiotherapy to take place, which is beneficial remains unresolved.

Stimulation Produced Analgesia

Acupuncture. Electroacupuncture was used to treat successfully 14 of 20 patients with established RSD in one uncontrolled series (13). All patients had received analgesics and physiotherapy for at least one month prior to treatment. The authors suggest that the decrease in pain associated with the electroacupuncture was responsible for the increased muscle power experienced by the majority of their patients. There was little or no improvement in range of movement in the affected limb.

TENS (Transcutaneous electrical nerve stimulation. TENS has been used for some time to treat RSD, but published results are rare. The mechanism of action remains unclear although Meyer and Fields felt that selective large fibre activity was responsible for the clinical effect in their study of eight patients (26). Two of the patients in this study were much better after treatment, 4 obtained transient relief and 2 were unchanged. TENS has been used successfully to treat RSD in adults (27) and 3 children; occasioning 3 reports (28-30).

The effect of TENS on the sympathetic nervous system has been studied following the initial report of Abram of an apparent increase in sympathetic activity and the development of RSD with repeated use of TENS to treat a neuroma (31). Further studies suggested that TENS did not alter cutaneous temperature, pulse rate, blood pressure, pupil size or skin impedance in either patients with chronic pain or controls (32). However, a later study showed a rise in skin temperature when infrared thermography was used (33).

TENS has been used experimentally. Procacci and his colleagues have recorded skin potentials, sensory thresholds and electromyelographic responses in affected extremities and conclude that the severity of the involvement correlates with the degree of sensory threshold depression (34).

Drug Therapy

Adrenergic blocking drugs. The apparently successful treatment of RSD by adrenergic blocking drugs such as guanethidine given by intravenous regional technique has prompted others to try many drugs in a similar fashion. Bretylium, reserpine, hydralazine, thymoxamine, phenoxybenzamine, phentolamine, methyldopa, clonidine, naftidrofuryl, droperidol and even lysine acetylsalicylate have been used with varying degrees of success. Thus it would appear logical to try the systemic use of both alpha- and beta- adrenergic blocking drugs. Unfortunately, clinical trials of these drugs have met with limited success, despite several papers that claim outstanding results. This disappointing state of affairs probably reflects differences in the mechanisms of the many conditions that are known as "reflex sympathetic dystrophy." However, there are reasonable grounds for believing that there may be a role for these agents in the management of RSD.

Alpha-adrenergic blocking drugs. Afferent fibres ending in an experimental neuroma have been shown to develop alpha-adrenergic sensitivity (35), and a response to sympathetic stimulation (36). This action would account for the relief of pain seen with alpha-blocking drug such as phenoxybenzamine, phentolamine, and prazocin. Further evidence to support the role of noradrenaline can be obtained from the increase in pain seen with the injection of noradrenaline in patients who have been relieved of pain by sympathectomy (37).

Phenoxybenzamine is a postsynaptic alpha-1 and presynaptic alpha-2 blocking drug. Ghostine and co-workers reported an uncontrolled series of 40 patients successfully treated with increasing daily doses of 40 to 120 mg of this drug (38). Duration of treatment was 6 to 8 weeks and local resolution of pain was achieved in all cases. Phentolamine has similar actions to phenoxybenzamine and has been used as treatment (39), and also to predict the response to oral prazocin, a relatively selective alpha-1 adrenergic blocker (40,41).

The mixed alpha- and beta-blocking drug labetalol has been used successfully in an intravenous regional technique (42), but there are no reports of systemic use to date.

Beta-adrenergic blocking drugs. There are isolated case reports of the successful use of propranolol (24,43,44), and an equally isolated report of failure (45). The presumed mechanism is blockade of the pre-junctional beta-2 receptor which will cause release of noradrenaline if stimulated (46).

Ketanserin. There are open studies reporting the successful use of this serotonin antagonist in the treatment of causalgia (47,48). An intravenous regional technique was followed by oral therapy of up to 80 mg daily in divided doses.

Calcium-channel blocking drugs. Initial studies with these agents are in progress. In theory, these agents should have a beneficial effect as sympathomimetic amines depend upon calcium flux for their action. The alpha-adrenergic stimulation with noradrenaline produces peripheral vasoconstriction secondary to increased calcium entry and increased calcium mobilisation in vascular smooth muscle cells. The beta-adrenergic agonists augment the calcium influx by increasing the number of functional calcium channels. There are data which suggest that hypercalcaemia may stimulate both alpha- and beta-adrenergic receptors although the results are variable.

Non-steroidal anti-inflammatory drugs [NSAIDs]. This large group of drugs are cited as being useful in the early treatment of RSD (49,50). However, the references quoted to justify these statements do not mention their use. NSAIDs were used with physiotherapy in the successful treatment of mild cases of RSD reported by Swezey (51).

Corticosteroids. Early reports of the use of steroids in the management of shoulder hand syndrome (52-54), were followed by a series of patients with RSD (55). Seventeen patients were treated with 20 mg of prednisone daily for an average of 26 weeks. Excellent results were claimed for 41%, good to fair for 35%, and poor results in 24%. Kozin and colleagues have published two papers reporting the use of high dose prednisone in RSD (56,57).

These series are not controlled, nor do all the patients satisfy the criteria for RSD, as three of the most important features; burning pain, hyperpathia, and response to sympathetic block were not present in some patients. Eighty-two percent of those who did satisfy the diagnostic criteria had good or excellent responses to systemic corticosteroids. There was no relationship between the duration of symptoms and the clinical response, and many of the cases were of over 6 months duration.

A more recent paper employed a randomised, placebo- controlled design to study the effects of 30 mg. of prednisone daily in divided doses. The study was continued until clinical resolution or 12 weeks. Improvement was seen in all the prednisone at the end of the trial, with only 20% of the placebo group showing any improvement (58). Steroids have also been employed in a regional intravenous technique (59).

The mechanisms by which steroids help RSD are unclear. They may stabilise basement membranes and reduce capillary permeability, thereby decreasing the plasma extravasation associated with the early stages of the disease. However, this does not explain the apparent success of this sort of treatment in established cases.

Other Drugs

Many other drugs have been tried in the management of RSD. There are theoretical reasons to believe that the alpha-adrenergic blocking actions of neuroleptic drugs such as chlorpromazine and haloperidol may be beneficial (60), but droperidol was unsuccessful when used in an intravenous regional technique (61). Antidepressives and anxiolytics have been employed for some time as analgesics rather than to control the emotional component (62), however, there are no adequate controlled studies to document any benefit, and at least one author believes their use is more out of desperation than because of widespread therapeutic success (63).

The same situation applies to the use of anticonvulsants where there are theoretical grounds for believing that they may be useful to control any lancinating or paroxysmal component to the pain. There is a case report of the successful use of phenytoin (64).

Use of calcitonin has been mentioned, but without comment as to its efficacy (65). The enkephalinase inhibitor D-phenylalanine has also been used empirically, but no results were given (66).

Summary

Successful treatment of reflex sympathetic dystrophy is directed at the restoration of normal function. Initial treatment should concentrate on management of the precipitating injury if necessary. Thereafter, there is general agreement that physiotherapy is a vital part of any treatment programme. It is a matter of regret that there are almost no adequate controlled studies of any type of non-invasive therapy. Future studies must concern themselves with the sort of physiotherapy to be applied and to identifying those measures that are most appropriate to judge treatment progress and outcome.

Other non-invasive techniques such as stimulation-produced analgesia and pharmacology, particularly the use of adrenergic blocking agents, hold some promise of future benefit. Here too, more effort should be made to carry out properly designed studies, as there is skepticism about the place of permanent or potentially destructive therapy in any painful condition. If the underlying mechanism for pain is one of neural damage, it is difficult to believe that matters can be improved by doing more damage.

REFERENCES

1. Sunderland, S. Nerves and nerve injuries, 2nd edn. Edinburgh, Churchill Livingstone, 1978.

2. Bonica, J.J. Causalgia and other reflex sympathetic dystrophies. In: Bonica, J. J., Liebeskind, J. C., Albe-Fessard, D. [eds.] Advances in Pain Research and Therapy, Vol. 3, New York, Raven Press, pp. 141-166, 1978.

3. Roberts, W.J. An hypothesis on the physiological basis for causalgia and related pains. Pain, 24: 297-311, 1986.

4. Schott, G.D. Mechanisms of causalgia and related clinical conditions: the role of the central and the sympathetic nervous systems. Brain, 109: 717-738, 1986.

5. McQuay, H.J., Carroll, D., Moore, R.A. Postoperative orthopaedic pain the effect of opiate premedication and local anaesthetic blocks. Pain, 33: 291-296, 1988.

6. Bach, S., Noreng, M.F., Tjellden, N.U. Phantom limb pain in amputees during the first twelve months following limb amputation, after preoperative lumbar epidural blockade. Pain, 33: 297-302, 1988.

7. Wall, P.D. The prevention of postoperative pain. Pain, 33: 289-290, 1988.

8. Baker, E.G., Winegarner, F.G. Causalgia: A review of 28 treated cases. Am J Surg, 117: 690-694, 1969.

9. Omer, G., Thomas, S. Treatment of causalgia: review of cases at Brooke General Hospital. Texas Med. 67: 63-67, 1971.

10. Pak, T.J. et al. Reflex sympathetic dystrophy: review of 140 cases. Minn Med. 53: 507-512, 1970.

11. Lindblom, U. Neuralgia: mechanisms and therapeutic prospects. In: Benedetti, C., Chapman, C.R., Morrica, G. [eds.] Advances in Pain Research and Therapy, Vol 7. Raven Press, New York. pp. 427-436, 1984.

12. Mitchell, S.W. Injuries of nerves and their consequences. Lippincott, New York, 1872.

13. Chan, C.S., Chow, S.P. Electroacupuncture in the treatment of posttraumatic sympathetic dystrophy [Sudeck's Atrophy]. Brit. J. Anaesth. 53: 899-902, 1981.

14. Frost, S.A. et al. Does hyperalgesia to cooling stimuli characterize patients with sympathetically maintained pain [reflex sympathetic dystrophy]? In: Dubner, R. Gebhart, G.F., Bond, M.R. [eds.] Proceedings of the Vth World Congress on Pain. Amsterdam, Elsevier, pp. 151-156, 1988.

15. Lehman, J. [ed.]. Therapeutic heat and cold. 4th edn. Baltimore, Williams and Wilkins, 1988.

16. Schumacher, H.B., Abramson, D.I. Post-traumatic vasomotor disorders: with particular reference to late manifestations and treatment. Surg. Gynecol Obstet., 88: 417-434, 1949.

17. Berstein, B.H., Singsen, B.H., Kent, J.T. Reflex neurovascular dystrophy in childhood. J. Pediatr., 93: 211-215, 1978.

18. Kim, H.J., Kozin, F., Johnson, R.P. Reflex sympathetic dystrophy syndrome of the knee following meniscectomy. Arthritis Rheum, 22: 177-181, 1979.

19. Goodman, C.R. Treatment of shoulder hand syndrome. Combined ultrasonic application to stellate ganglion and physical medicine. N.Y. State J. Med., 71: 559-562, 1971.

20. Johnson, E.W., Pannazzo, A.N. Management of shoulder hand syndrome. J Amer Med Ass, 193:152-154, 1966.

21. Fermaglich, D.R. Reflex sympathetic dystrophy in children. Pediatrics, 60: 881-883, 1977.

22. Wettrell, G., Hallbook, T., Hultquist, C. Reflex sympathetic dystrophy in two young females. Acta Pediatr. Scand., 68: 923-924, 1979.

23. Goldner, J.L. Cause and prevention of reflex sympathetic dystrophy. J. Hand Surg. 5: 295-296, 1980.

24. Visitsunthorn, U., Prete, P. Reflex sympathetic dystrophy of the lower extremity: a complication of herpes zoster with dramatic response to propranolol. West. J. Med., 135: 62-66, 1981.

25. Kleinert, H.E., et al. Post-traumatic reflex sympathetic dystrophy. Orthop. Clin. North Am., 4: 917-925, 1973.

26. Meyer, G.A., Fields, H.L. Causalgia treated by selective large fibre stimulation of peripheral nerve. Brain, 95: 163-166, 1972.

27. Bohm, E. TENS in chronic pain after peripheral nerve injury. Acta Neurosurg. [Wien.], 40: 277-285, 1978.

28. Stilz, R.J., Carron, H., Sanders D.B. Reflex sympathetic dystrophy in a six year old. Successful treatment by transcutaneous nerve stimulation. Anesth. Analg. 56: 438-443, 1977.

29. Richlin, D.M. et al. Reflex sympathetic dystrophy: successful treatment by transcutaneous nerve stimulation. J. Pediatr., 93: 84-86, 1978.

30. Leo, K.C. Use of electrical stimulation at acupuncture points for the treatment of reflex sympathetic dystrophy in a child. Phys. Ther., 63: 957-959, 1983.

31. Abram. S.E. Increased sympathetic tone associated with TENS. Anesthesiology, 45: 575-577, 1976.

32. Ebersold, M.J., Laws, E.R., Albers, J.W. Measurement of autonomic function before during and after transcutaneous stimulation in patients with chronic pain and control subjects. Mayo Clin. Proc., 52: 228-232, 1977.

33. Owens, S., Atkinson, E.R., Lees, D.E. Thermographic evidence of reduced sympathetic tone with transcutaneous nerve stimulation. Anesthesiology, 50: 62-65, 1970.

34. Procacci, P. et al. Skin potential and EMG changes induced by cutaneous electrical stimulation. II. Subjects with reflex sympathetic dystrophies. Appl. Neurophysiol., 42: 125-134, 1979.

35. Wall, P.D., Gutnick, M. Ongoing activity in peripheral nerves. the physiology and pharmacology of impulses originating from a neuroma. Exp. Neurol., 43: 580-593, 1974.

36. Devor, M., Janig, W. Activation of myelinated afferents ending in a neuroma by stimulation of the sympathetic supply in the rat. Neurosci Lett., 24: 43-47, 1981.

37. Wiesenfeld-Hallin, Z., Hallin, R.G. The influence of the sympathetic system on mechanoreception and nociception. A review. Hum. Neurobiol., 3: 41-46, 1984.

38. Ghostine, S.Y. et al. Phenoxybenzamine in the treatment of causalgia. J Neurosurg., 60: 1263-1268, 1984.

39. Campbell, J.N., Raja, S.N., Meyer, R.A. Painful sequelae of nerve injury. In: Dubner, R., Gebhart, G.F. Bond, M.R. [eds.], Proceedings of the Vth World congress on Pain. Amsterdam, Elsevier, pp. 135-143, 1986.

40. Abram, S.E., Lightfoot, R. Treatment of longstanding causalgia with prazocin. Reg. Anesth., 6: 79-81, 1981.

41. Abram, S.E. Pain of sympathetic origin. In: Raj, P.P. [ed.], Practical Management of Pain. Chicago, Year Book Medical Publishers. pp. 451-463, 1986.

42. Parris, W.C.V., Harris, R., Lindsey, K. Use of intravenous regional labetalol in treating resistant reflex sympathetic dystrophy. Pain Suppl., 4: S206, 1987.

43. Simson, C. Propranolol for causalgia and Sudeck's atrophy. J. Amer. Med. Ass., 227: 327, 1974.

44. Pleet, A.R., Tahmoush, A.J., Jennings, J.R. Causalgia. Treatment with propranolol. Neurology [Minneap.], 26: 375, 1976.

45. Magee, J. Propranolol for causalgia and Sudeck's atrophy. J. Amer. Med. Ass., 228: 826-827, 1974.

46. Stjarne, L., Brundin, J. Beta-2 adrenoreceptors facilitate noradrenaline release from human vasoconstrictor fibres. Acta Physiol. Scand., 97: 88-93, 1976.

47. Moesker, A. et al. Treatment of post-traumatic dystrophy [Sudeck's atrophy] with guanethidine and ketanserin. Pain Clin., 1: 171-176, 1985.

48. Davies, J.A.H., Beswick, T., Dickson, G. Ketanserin and guanethidine in the treatment of causalgia. Anesth Analg., 66: 575-576, 1987.

49. Schwartzman, R.J., McLellan T.L. Reflex sympathetic dystrophy, a review. Arch. Neurol., 44: 555-561, 1987.

50. Casey, K.L. Toward a rationale for the treatment of painful neuropathies. In: Dubner, R., Gebhart, G.F. Bond, M.R. [eds.], Proceedings of the Vth World congress on Pain. Amsterdam, Elsevier, pp. 165-174. 1986.

51. Swezey, R.L. Transient, osteoporosis of the hip, foot and knee. Arthritis Rheum., 13: 858-868, 1970.

52. Steinbrocker, O., Neustadt, D., Lapin, L. Shoulder hand syndrome: Sympathetic block compared with corticotrophin and cortisone therapy. JAMA, 153: 788-791, 1946.

53. Russek, H.I. et al. Cortisone in the treatment of shoulder-hand syndrome following acute myocardial infarction. Arch. Int. Med., 91: 487-492, 1953.

54. Russek, H.I. Shoulder-hand syndrome following myocardial infarction. Med Clin. North Am., 42: 1555-1562, 1958.

55. Glick, E.N. Reflex dystrophy [algoneurodystrophy]. Results of treatment by corticosteroids. Rheumatol. Rehab., 12: 84-88, 1973.

56. Kozin, F. et al. The reflex sympathetic dystrophy syndrome. I. Clinical and histologic studies: Evidence for bilaterality, response to corticosteroids and articular involvement. Am. J. Med., 60: 321-331, 1976.

57. Kozin, F. et al. The reflex sympathetic dystrophy syndrome. III. Scintigraphic studies, further evidence for the therapeutic activity of systemic corticosteroids, and proposed diagnostic criteria. Am. J. Med., 70: 23-30, 1981.

58. Christensen, K. Jensen, E.M., Noer, I. The reflex sympathetic dystrophy syndrome; response to treatment with systemic corticosteroids. Acta Chir. Scand., 148: 653-655, 1982.

59. Poplawski, Z.J., Wiley, A.M., Murray, J.F. Post-traumatic dystrophy of the extremities. A clinical review and trial of treatment. J. Bone and Jt. Surg., 65-A: 642-655, 1983.

60. Kocher, R. Use of psychotrophic drugs for the treatment of chronic severe pain. In: Bonica, J.J. Albe-Fessard, D. [eds.], Advances in Pain Research and Therapy, Vol. 1. New York, Raven Press, pp. 579-582, 1976.

61. Kettler, R.E., Abram, S.E. Intravenous regional droperidol in the management of reflex sympathetic dystrophy: A double blind, placebo-controlled, crossover study. Anesthesiology, 69: 933-936, 1988.

62. Taub, A., Collins, W.F. Observations on the treatment of denervation dysesthesia with psychotrophic drugs: Postherpetic neuralgia, anesthesia dolorosa, peripheral neuropathy. In: bonica, J.J. [ed.], Advances in Neurology, Vol 4. New York, Raven Press, pp. 309-315. 1974.

63. Rowlingson, J.C. The sympathetic dystrophies. Int. Anesth. Clinics, 21[4]: 117-129, 1983.

64. Chaturvedi, S.K. Phenytoin in reflex sympathetic dystrophy. Pain, 36: 379-380, 1989.

65. Editorial. Algodystrophy. Brit Med. J., i: 461-462, 1978.

66. Budd, K. Use of D-phenylalanine, an enkephalinase inhibitor, in the treatment of intractable pain. In: Bonica, J.J., Lindblom, U. Iggo. A. [eds.], Advances in Pain Research and Therapy, Vol. 5. New York, Raven Press, pp. 305-308, 1983.

17

MULTI-DISCIPLINARY MANAGEMENT OF REFLEX SYMPATHETIC DYSTROPHY

Prithvi Raj, Jeffrey Cannella, Jennifer Kelly,
Karen McConn, Patricia Lowry

The diagnosis and definition of reflex sympathetic dystrophy has already been well addressed in this text. It is also apparent from previous chapters that treatment is not always successful and that further comparative studies are required, in order to better our patient evaluation and treatment methods. A number of scales have also been proposed to confirm early diagnosis and initiate appropriate therapy (1,2). Although a small number of these cases of RSD obtain resolution spontaneously or with minimal therapy, most of those cases presenting to major treatment centers, suffer prolonged pain which is difficult or impossible to fully resolve.

This paper describes experience with a multi-disciplinary approach to treatment, based on a three week intensive inpatient program in order to bring patients to partial recovery, followed by outpatient therapy until full relief and function is restored.

METHOD

Patient Assessment

A total of 23 patients with RSD have participated in this program to date. Their sex and age distribution, nature and duration of injury, are presented in Table 1. Clinical grading scales were used to classify patients by severity of disease, using an array of symptoms, signs, test measures and 3 phase scintigraphy using the criteria of Demageat et al. (3), to derive one of three grades as presented in Table 2. In addition, twenty of this patient group received a further interview, MMPI evaluation (4) and Beck Hopelessness Scale (5), as part of a psychological assessment. These were used to help determine stressors related to the syndrome and evaluate the patients' coping mechanisms. The Hopelessness scale was sought as a measure of negative expectancies, to help obtain any correlation between this and outcome. The personality profile and evidence of stressors were used to help direct appropriate psychotherapy.

Functional evaluation involved testing the range of movement of the affected joints, using a 0-100 scale from no function to full function, muscle strength grading 1-5 by the method of manual muscle testing (6), and determination of an overall level of function score from 1-3. A score of 3 denoted no function, 2 was for function with assistance, and 1 represented full and normal function.

Table 1. Demographic Data

Number of Pts.	23
Male	12
Female	11
Age ≤ 35	14
≥ 35	9
Duration of Injury	
< 3 months	3
3-6 months	7
6-9 months	5
> 12 months	8
Type of Injury	
Soft tissue	15
Bone	5
Nerve injuries	2
Combined	1

Table 2. Reflex Sympathetic Dystrophy
Phases and Characteristics

	Phase I Acute	Phase II Dystrophic	Phase III Atrophic
PAIN	Burning/ Neuralgia + + +	Burning/ Throbbing + + + +	Burning/ Throbbing + +
DYSTHESIA	+ +	+ + +	+
FUNCTION	Minimal Impairment	Restricted	Severely Restricted
AUTONOMIC DYSFUNCTION	Increased Blood Flow	Normal or Decreased Flow	Decreased Blood Flow
TEMPERATURE	Increased	Decreased	Decreased
DISCOLORATION	Erythematous	Mottled/ Dusky	Cyanotic
SUDOMOTOR	Minimal	+ +	+ + +
EDEMA	+ +	+ + +	+
TROPHIC CHANGES	0	+ +	+ + + +
Nuclear Imaging (Scanning)			
Flow Phase	↑	-	↓
Pool Phase	↑	-	↓
Static Phase	↑		-

Treatment

Treatment was standardised according to protocol as shown in Table 3.

Table 3. RSD Therapeutic Regimen Protocol

I. Medications (oral) (daily)

    A. Analgesics (non-steroid anti-inflammatory agents, e.g., ibuprofen)
    B. Muscle relaxant (e.g., cyclobenzamine)
    C. Vasodilator (e.g., nifedipine)
    D. Antidepressant (e.g., amitriptyline)
    E. Hypnotic (e.g., chloral hydrate)

II. Regional Analgesic Technique
    (Intermittent or continuous) (daily)

    A. Upper extremity
      - Sympathetic block (stellate) or
      - Somatic block (brachial plexus or
        cervical epidural)
    B. Lower extremity
      - Sympathetic block (lumbar) or
      - Somatic block (lumbar epidural or sciatic)

III. Psychotherapy (twice a week)

    A. Cognitive coping strategies
    B. Biofeedback

IV. Physical Therapy (daily)

    A. Aggressive exercise program (passive, assisted, and active)
    B. Modality treatment (desensitization, deep heat, massage, etc.)

(Three week duration)

The regional anesthetic technique consisted of intermittent or continuous sympathetic blocks for 5 individuals, or somatic blocks (epidural or brachial plexus for the arm and sciatic for the leg), in the other 18. All but two patients received local anesthetic via continuous pump driven infusion, and all obtained adequate pain relief whether the block was continuous or intermittent.

Psychotherapy was provided in the form of cognitive coping strategies for 15 patients, two of whom also received biofeedback therapy.

Physical therapy consisted of aggressive daily exercises and some physical modalities (heat, ultrasound etc.) in all patients with continuous blocks, and twice weekly in the two patients having intermittent block analgesia.

OUTCOME

Because treatment in each case was continued to the point of functional and symptomatic resolution, outcome for the purpose of this report, was determined at the end of the three week aggressive therapy period. Responses at this time were graded as a rating of 1 for those patients with complete recovery; 2 for those still requiring assistance for their usual functions; 3 if there was no appreciable change from pre-treatment levels.

Overall, 14 patients had complete recovery at this time and 9 had partial recovery. Some remaining cases also recovered with time, but needed up to one and a half years of treatment before recovery was complete.

Clinical phasing of the 23 patients showed different grading on clinical compared to radiological criteria. Assignment on clinical grounds to either of phases I, II, or III, was for 6, 10, and 7 cases respectively; on 3 phase scintigraphy these numbers were 9, 2, and 5, with a further 5 patients having normal scans despite a clinical grading into phases II or III, and two patients were not studied, i.e., scanning changes are not specific for RSD diagnosis, though it may help identify early cases. (See the next chapter for more specific detail.) There was no significant difference in outcome dependent on phasing in these grades. The results indicated that younger patients showed better outcome than did those over 35 years, ($p = < 0.05$). In this small series, the nature of the patient's injury was not a discriminating factor in outcome.

Psychological evaluation was primarily intended to define patient profiles. Two-thirds of the patients exhibited elevation in MMPI profiles in at least one scale, with females and younger patients under 35, showing significantly higher scores in either F, paranoia, and depression scales. The discriminate analysis further revealed that treatment outcome was better for those patients with higher hypomanic and masculinity-femininity scales, p= <.05. The Beck Hopelessness scales proved essentially normal and were of no value in predicting outcome, but patients receiving workers compensation benefits did have significantly higher scores as determined by an analysis of variance (p= <.01). This indicates that those on workers compensation benefits were more pessimistic, though it did not apparently influence outcome.

Treatment variables showed no difference in outcome between either the sympathetic or somatic block techniques in deriving improvement. However, with only 5 patients in the sympathetic block group, the numbers may not be sufficient to reveal any distinction. It is also likely that with the somatic nerve blocks provided, there would also be a component of sympathetic block as part of this therapy. A majority of patients received multiple medications as contained in the treatment protocol.

Functional disability responses measuring range of motion, muscle strength, and total functional level, were compared from pre- to post-treatment scores, and are depicted as percentage changes in Figure 1. All measures showed considerable and significant improvement.

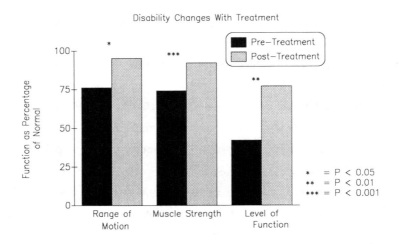

Figure 1. Disability changes with treatment

DISCUSSION

Sustained and adequate pain relief seems to be one of the important factors in managing and resolving RSD (7). This allows the institution of aggressive care, particularly exercise therapy, in conjunction with a multimodal approach, in order to resolve the physical and psychological disability associated with RSD. The majority of patients in this study required continuous somatic rather than the tradition sympathetic block, in order to obtain a satisfactory level of pain relief. Provision of this somewhat new approach to analgesia was deemed necessary because previous sympathetic blocks had been inadequate in these same patients. Failure of sympathetic block, despite a diagnosis of reflex sympathetic dystrophy on clinical and radiological criteria, may only imply that pain is still arising from other somatic sources as well. Failure of symptomatic relief with sympathetic block does not preclude a diagnosis of sympathetic dystrophy, though positive responses as described by Boas in Chapter 11 are still required to sustain the diagnosis. It may also be that the use of somatic blocks also obscured any difference in outcome, as is usually the case, due to differences in the nature of underlying causes, such as soft tissue, bony or nerve injury.

It is difficult to determine positive conclusions from a small case series, but from the psychological profiles and the apparent difference in response from younger patients with a shorter time interval between injury and treatment, it would appear that RSD has a two phase presentation. It seems that RSD may be a syndrome which has an acute severe phase, followed by course of prolonged rehabilitation. It is during the rehabilitation period that patients show chronic pain behaviour.

An early aggressive multi-disciplinary treatment program as presented offers better pain relief and rapid improvement in function, so that patients do not enter the phase of a chronic pain syndrome. We do not share the view of some clinicians, who believe that dramatic relief and cure for reflex sympathetic dystrophy can be sustained by any single mode of therapy used in isolation.

REFERENCES

1. Low, P.A., Caskey, P.E., Tuck, P.R., Fealey, R.D., Dyck, P.J. Quantitative sudomotor axon reflex test in normal and neuropathic subjects. Ann. Neurol., 14: 573-580, 1983.

2. Wilson, P.R. Sympathetically-maintained pain. In Stanton-Hicks, M. (ed.), Pain and the Sympathetic Nervous System. Kluwer Academic Publishers, Norwell, MA, 1989.

3. Demageat, J.L. et al. Three phase bone scanning in reflex sympathetic dystrophy of the hand. J. Nucl. Med., 29: 26-32, 1987.

4. Greene, R.L. The MMPI: An Interpretative Manual. Grune and Stratton, New York, 1980.

5. Beck, A.T., Weissman, A., Lester, D., Trexler, L. The measure of hopelessness: The hopelessness scale. J. Couns. Clin. Psychol., 42: 861-865, 1974.

6. Daniels, L. Muscle testing: Techniques of manual exam. 2nd ed. W. B. Saunders, Philadelphia, 1975.

7. Cooper, D.E., DeLee, J.C., Ramamurthy, S.A. Reflex sympathetic dystrophy of the knee. J. Bone and Joint Surg., 71A: 365-369, 1989.

SUMMARY OF SECTION III

THERAPEUTIC TECHNIQUES IN RSD

Technical issues relating to conduct of intravenous blocks dominated in the first instance. Use of an initial regional anesthetic block of the sympathetic ganglion or somatic nerves of the affected limb was felt appropriate in very severe pain states, where tourniquets, needles and exsanguination were not tolerated. Distal venous injection was felt preferable in order to reduce risks of leak into the systemic circulation. Reiteration of the role of sympathetic blocks focused discussion around their capacity to allow reactivation and exercise as their primary function. Previously the literature emphasis on sympathectomy as a treatment in itself has probably been the basis for many failed treatments. Neurolytic blocks were not thought appropriate in this context because they tend not to be permanent as had been thought because the induced scarring about ganglia might preclude complete solution spread in any future blocks, notwithstanding a small number of patients with intractable symptoms who may respond successfully to a neurolytic sympathectomy.

Temperature measurement at distal digital skin sites was considered a simple, specific and cost effective monitor for both diagnosis and treatment response assessment.

Section IV

NEW TECHNIQUES

18

THREE-PHASE BONE SCANNING IN REFLEX SYMPATHETIC DYSTROPHY

H. Steinert, O. Nickel, K. Hahn

Since the introduction of 99m-Technetium-Phosphonate in bone scanning techniques, several researchers have reported their experiences with three-phase bone scanning in RSD. Kozin et al. (1) compared radiographs and scintigraphy, assessing their sensitivity and specificity with RSD patients. A comparison of sensitivity and specificity revealed that sensitivity assessed by scintigraphy gave similar results to those observed with radiography (60% vs. 69%), while specificity was distinctly higher (92% vs. 79%), suggesting that this would be an important aid in the diagnosis of reflex sympathetic dystrophy.

Holder and Mackinnon (2) investigated sensitivity and specificity during the three different scan phases. Sensitivity during phases 1 and 2 was low, 45% and 52%, while it ranged to 96% during phase 3. Specificity of all three phases was very high (between 94% and 98%). Demangeat (3) performed scintigraphy in 181 patients with RSD of the hand. Using different parameters it was possible to identify three stages of RSD as follows: 1. stage: 0-20 weeks, 2. stage: 20-60 weeks, 3. stage: 60-100 weeks. A comparison of the data obtained by the different researchers shows that, at the time of the radionuclide investigation, a clinical diagnosis of RSD was available. At present no studies investigating the differentiation between RSD and simple inactivity osteoporosis have been attempted.

The scintigraphic studies already published do not permit valid comparisons due to the use of different types of equipment and varying time frame protocols employed for the angiogram. For these reasons a more specific and precise method has been developed and is described.

METHOD

The patient is placed in front of a large field of view gamma camera (Figure 1) with his hands placed palms down on the surface of a special high-sensitivity, parallel-hole collimator. A bolus injection is made through a contralateral antecubital vein by using a special catheter system (Figure 2). At first a 0.3-0.5 ml solution, containing up to 15 mCi 99m-Tc-DPD, is injected into the catheter. This injection is followed by rapidly flushing 20 ml of saline solution (8 ml/sec) to get a compact bolus.

Sixty, 2 second-frames are acquired starting at the time of intravenous injection. These images show the bolus of activity passing through the radial and ulnar arteries. The flow through the palmar arches is seen as a blush. Activity in the fingers normally appears either in the same frame as the palmar arches or in the next frame.

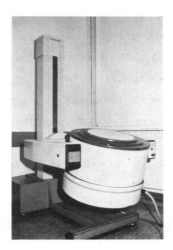

Figure 1. Gamma camera

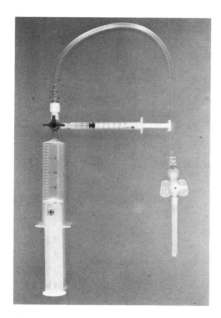

Figure 2. Catheter system

INTERPRETATION

In the sequential study presented (Figure 3), the arterial blood flow is a little delayed in the left hand. (This is not typical for RSD.)

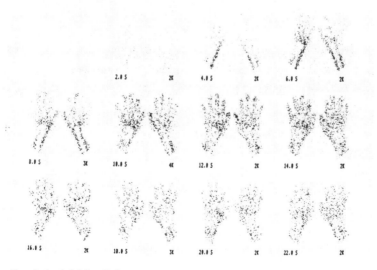

Figure 3. Arterial blood flow

When this dynamic series of frames has been recorded, a static 200 sec frame is obtained immediately--without moving the patient's hands. In this phase the radio nuclide is in equilibrium with the vascular and interstitial compartment, the blood pool images show the relative vascularisation of the soft tissues. Figure 4 shows a slight hyperemia in the left hand and in some juxta-articular regions of the fingers.

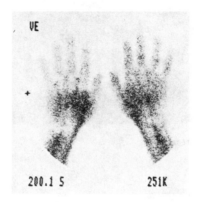

Figure 4. Soft tissue vascularization

Three hours after injection, soft tissue activity has cleared substantially. Now the so-called "delayed" static images are taken with a high resolution collimator. These images demonstrate the bone metabolism.

Figure 5 shows a diffusely increased uptake in all juxta-articular regions of all joints of the left hand. This patient suffered from a soft tissue injury of his left hand; the bone scan demonstrates an osteoporosis resulting from immobilization.

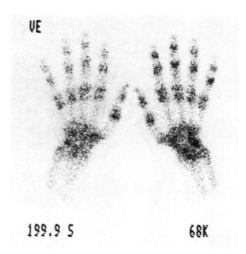

Figure 5.

An example of RSD in Stage I is demonstrated by the blood flow study and delayed image. The flow is diffusely increased in all parts of the wrist and hand; increased perfusion can also be seen in the radial and ulnar arteries. The delayed image shows the typically increased uptake in the periarticular regions of the affected hand (Figures 6,7,8).

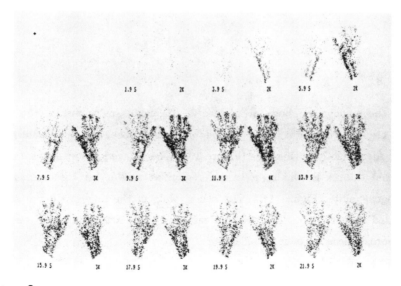

Figure 6.

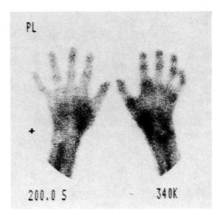

Figure 7.

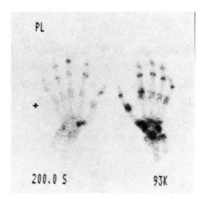

Figure 8.

In the angiogram shown in Figure 9, the perfusion seems to stop in the carpal region of the right hand. In the following frames, a hypervascularisation can be seen exactly in this area (Figure 10). The delayed image shows a diffuse increased uptake in the right carpal region as well as in three metacarpophalangeal joints (Figure 11). The other joints of the fingers show a slightly increased activity too. This patient suffered from arthritis and a resulting osteoporosis because of immobilisation.

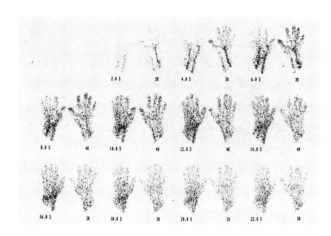

Figure 9.

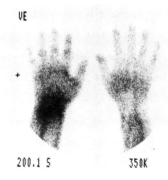

Figure 10.

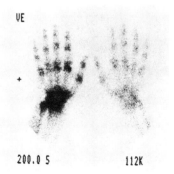

Figure 11.

It is possible to evaluate regional blood flow using first circulation time-activity curves. These diagrams can be constructed by drawing regions of interest on equal parts of both hands during first circulation. Time-activity curves always show two different phases during the first minutes after bolus injection: 1) the inflow phase during first pass, and 2) the stable equilibration phase after one minute.

The RSD-patient shows an earlier and higher increase of the arterial inflow in the affected hand. This is the typical pattern of the first pass of RSD-patients in the initial stage.

DEVELOPMENT

Although not widely recognized, it has been shown mathematically that first circulation time-activity curves reflect two physiologic parameters: 1) the relative mean transit time from the injection site to and through the regions of interest, and 2) the relative blood volume (4). These parameters can be used to evaluate regional blood flow.

The regional blood volume is determined from the integral of the first pass. For precise mathematical calculation, extrapolation of the first pass curve beyond the point of recirculation is necessary (see Figure 12). This requires special computer software.

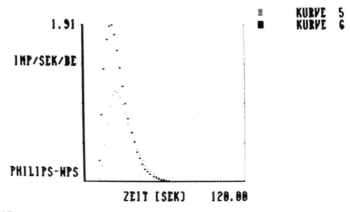

Figure 12.

The measurement of blood volume is generally expressed as a ratio in terms of the volume of the vascular space relative to the volume of the region rather than a unitary volume. In general, the volume of the vascular space is unknown and cannot be determined easily.

Blood flow is not uniquely determined by mean transit time and blood volume. We have to take into account that the tracer flows after the intravenous injection through the right heart, the lung, and the left heart. The lung uptake and the cardiac output therefore influence the blood flow.

Much more work is required to obtain a clinically useful method for quantification of blood flow. Use of a gamma camera and scintillation probes will shortly assist in this end by allowing measurement of cardiac output.

REFERENCES

1. Kozin, F. et al. Bone scintigraphy in the reflex sympathetic dystrophy syndrome. Radiology, 138: 437-443, 1981.

2. Holder, L.E., Mackinnon, S.E. Reflex sympathetic dystrophy in the hands: Clinical and scintigraphic criteria. Radiology, 152: 517-522, 1984.

3. Demangeat, J.L. et al. Three-phase bone scanning in reflex sympathetic dystrophy of the hand. J Nucl Med, 29: 26-32, 1987.

4. Klingensmith, W.C. Physiologic interpretation of time-activity curves from cerebral flow studies: Theoretical considerations. J Nucl Med All Sci, 24: 73-78, 1980.

19

AN INVESTIGATION OF THE ROLE OF CLONIDINE
IN THE TREATMENT OF REFLEX SYMPATHETIC DYSTROPHY

Chris J. Glynn, Peter C. Jones

INTRODUCTION

The possible central and spinal mechanisms involved in the transmission of the pain of reflex sympathetic dystrophy (RSD) are discussed in detail in this volume. This study is designed to investigate the possible mechanisms involved in the transmission of pain of RSD at the postganglionic synapse. Guanethidine has been used successfully to treat the pain of RSD as described by Hannington-Kiff (Chapter 12) and (1). This pain relief has been shown to be associated with sympathetic blockade as measured by an increase in skin blood flow, and abolition of the vasoconstrictor ice response (2). Thus the pain relief achieved with this technique is believed, in part, to be a result of sympathetic blockade at the postganglionic synapse, indicating a possible role for the synapse in pain transmission.

RSD most commonly results from trauma in the periphery, and so it is reasonable to assume that some "cause" of the pain may also be in the periphery. This study investigated the role of clonidine, an alpha 2 agonist, given via an intravenous regional (Bier's block) in the treatment of pain in this patient group.. Thus it was possible to compare the effect of guanethidine, (a false transmitter of noradrenalin) to clonidine, (blocking presynaptic release of noradrenalin) in the same patient.

PATIENTS AND METHODS

Twenty-two patients agreed to participate in the study, which had approval of the local Ethics Committee. There were 13 females and 9 males. The diagnosis of RSD was made in these patients on clinical grounds, and confirmed by 24 hours of pain relief following guanethidine block, suggesting an involvement of the sympathetic nervous system in the transmission of each patient's pain. Nineteen patients had RSD of various causes (Table 1), 2 had Rheumatoid Arthritis (RA), and 1 had Post-Herpetic Neuralgia (PHN). The mean age of the patients was 54 years with a range of 30-87 years. The mean duration of pain was 45 months with a range from 3 to 240 months. After previous positive responses to guanethidine block, clonidine 150ug in 10ml of physiological saline was compared in a double-blind random fashion to 10ml of physiological saline given intravenously as a Bier's block (4) to the affected limb, on 2 separate occasions at least a week apart. The ice response to skin blood flow was measured by venous occlusion plethysmography (3,5) with a mercury strain gauge on the thumbs or great toes before and after each injection. Pain intensity, pain relief, and mood were assessed by using the visual analogue scale before and after the injection, and again half an hour later just prior to discharge. Blood pressure was also measured manually at the same times, and any other comments by the patient about either injection were recorded. The effect of each injection on the somatic nervous system was assessed before discharge by sensory (pinprick) and motor (power) testing.

TABLE 1.

No.	Sex	Age	Diagnosis	Duration of Pain in Months	Oral Clonidine
1.	F	71	RSD L foot PS	36	yes
2.	F	70	RSD L foot PS	18	yes
3.	M	46	RSD R hand PS	22	no
4.	M	56	RSD L hand SY	120	yes
5.	M	53	RSD L hand PS	7	yes
6.	F	76	RSD L hand PS	8	yes
7.	F	30	RSD L foot PS	30	yes
8.	F	55	RSD L foot PS	16	yes
9.	F	57	RSD R foot PS	240	yes
10.	F	87	RSD L foot I	6	no
11.	F	46	RSD R hand PS	12	no
12.	M	32	RSD R foot PT	10	no
13.	F	46	RSD L hand PS	12	no
14.	M	42	RSD R hand PT	14	no
15.	M	45	RSD R hand PT	3	yes
16.	M	42	RSD R hand PT	13	yes
17.	M	76	PHN R hand	24	?
18.	F	57	RA L hand	120	?
19.	F	40	RSD R hand PS	24	yes
20.	F	57	RA L foot	120	?
21.	M	51	RSD R hand SY	102	yes
22.	F	56	RSD R hand I	30	no

RSD = Reflex Sympathetic Dystrophy, RA = Rheumatoid Arthritis, PHN = Post-Herpetic Neuralgia, PS = Post- Surgical, PT = Posttraumatic, I = Idiopathic, and SY = Syringomyelia

Statistical Analyses

The Wilcoxon matched pairs tests for small samples has been used throughout, a result will only be considered significant if p < 0.012, assuming an average correlation of 0.5.

RESULTS

Pain and Mood

Although clonidine decreased the reported pain intensity more than placebo, when comparing the pre to the second post-injection recording, there was no statistical difference found between them (Figures 1-4). Neither was there any difference in pain relief scores and pain word scores. Clonidine was generally associated with a greater increase in the mood score (worse) than placebo but the difference was not statistically significant (Figures 5 and 6).

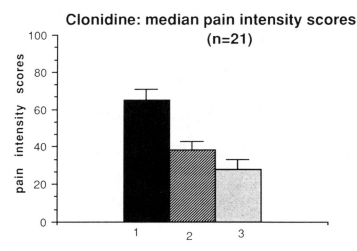

Figure 1.

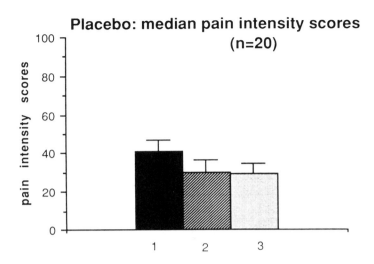

Figure 2.

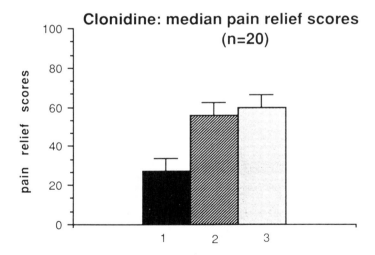

Figure 3.

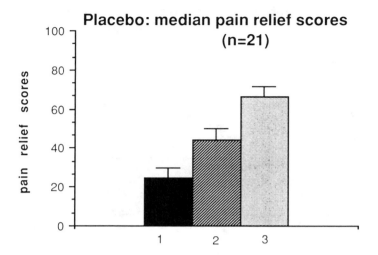

Figure 4.

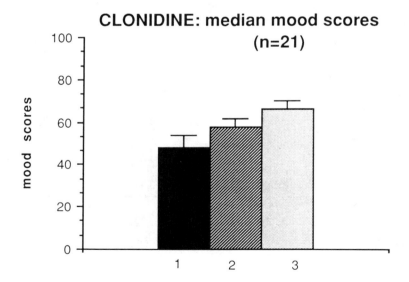

Figure 5.

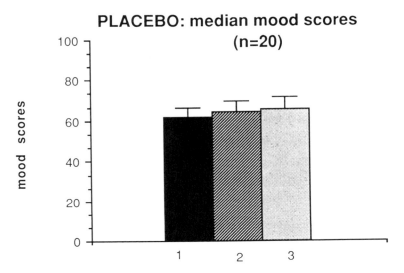

Figure 6.

Ice Response

All patients had a significant decrease in skin blood flow in both limbs following the application of ice to the neck before treatment with clonidine (p < 0.001). Following the block, this ice response disappeared in both the treated and the untreated groups. However, in those treated with saline there was a significant ice response (p < 0.001) in the treated limb, but not in the untreated limb (p < 0.07). This suggests that the tourniquet and/or the saline increased sympathetic activity in the treated limb.

Clinical Responses

Two patients (#12,15) obtained pain relief at the end of the study. Patient 12 required no further treatment, while patient 15 continued with oral clonidine for a month, and then ceased. Three patients (#19,21,22) who obtained relief, have continued with intermittent clonidine blocks, two (#21 22) taking additional oral clonidine. Two other patients (#1,8) are, two years later, still taking oral clonidine but obtain better relief with epidural rather than with Bier's block clonidine. One patient (#17) with post herpetic neuralgia, withdrew from the study after the first clonidine injection, because of pain aggravation, but his pain subsequently resolved spontaneously. Two patients (#18,20), both with rheumatoid arthritis, obtained lasting pain relief from the first injection. Patient 18 had clonidine, and patient 20 had saline. Four patients (#2,4,7,9) have obtained significant relief from a variety of other treatments. Three patients (#11, 13,16) continue to be difficult therapeutic problems. Five (#3,5,6,10,14) have been lost to follow-up. There was sensory or motor blockade following either injection, nor was there any significant hypotension.

Side-Effects

Four patients complained of side effects from the clonidine, three with dizziness (#6,9,10), and one with drowsiness (#14), while two patients complained of side effects from the saline, one with dizziness (#8), and one with depression (#16).

Discussion

Clonidine appears to have provided effective sympathetic blockade as measured by the diminished vasoconstrictor ice response, but without better analgesia when compared to placebo injection. This suggests that clonidine, an alpha 2 agonist or a pre-synaptic blocker of noradrenalin, blocks sympathetic transmission in the periphery, but not pain, when given via a Bier's block. This raises some questions in explanation of the peripheral mechanisms of RSD. It has been suggested that noradrenalin is a peripheral mediator of the pain of RSD (6), so that clonidine could be expected to relieve pain by preventing the release of noradrenalin; thus assuming such an effect was attained, it is possible that noradrenalin is not the important transmitter in RSD. But, guanethidine (a false transmitter of noradrenalin at the postganglionic synapse), was effective in providing pain relief in these patients. Three or more possible options may explain this difference: (i) The effect of guanethidine was a placebo response, similar to the saline placebo responses in the study; (ii) the responses were due to the effect of the tourniquet; (iii) there is a real difference between the effect of the two drugs. There is no way of excluding the first option without doing a placebo controlled study before the patients are admitted to the formal study. If this represents a tourniquet response, then it was probably not via sympathetic blockade because the placebo injection seemed to increase sympathetic activity as measured with an ice response. Thus it is possible that there was a real difference between the two drugs, but the design of the study was not powerful enough to identify this difference. Other methodological problems relating to the use of ice response testing and its interpretation, may also negate some of the conclusions.

Clinically, four patients still taking oral clonidine in migraine doses, are maintained with intermittent clonidine injections, two with Bier's blocks and two with epidural. Another was unable to take oral clonidine but obtains relief with intermittent Bier's blocks. Five patients recovered during the course of the study, but of these, one received saline and another withdrew as previously stated. Four patients are being successfully treated with a variety of other treatments. Eight of the patients failed to obtain any long-term benefit from clonidine.

In summary, Bier's block clonidine may have a limited place in the long-term treatment of some patients with RSD. Its use may be in the initial phase, allowing subsequent maintenance of relief with oral clonidine.

REFERENCES

1. Hannington-Kiff, J.G. Intravenous regional sympathetic block with guanethidine. Lancet, i: 1019-1020, 1974.
2. Glynn, C.J., Basedow, R.W., Walsh, J.A. Pain relief following postganglionic sympathetic blockade with intravenous guanethidine. Br. J. Anaesthesia, 53: 1297-1302, 1981.
3. Glynn, C.J., Walsh, J.A., Basedow, R.W., Marzola, M. A model for investigating the effect of drugs on the peripheral nervous system in man. J. Auto. Nervous System, 5: 195-205, 1981.

4. Bier, A. Veber einen neunen Weg Lokalanasthesie an den Giedmassen zu Erzeugen. Vertch. Dtsch. Ges. Chir., 37: 204, 1908.

5. Jamieson, G.G., Ludbrook, J., Wilson, A. The response of hand blood flow to distant ice application. Aust. J. exp. Biol. Med. Sci., 49: 145-152, 1971.

6. Roberts, W.J. A hypothesis on the physiological basis for causalgia and related pains. Pain, 24: 297-311, 1986.

SUMMARY OF SECTION IV

NEW TECHNIQUES

Discussions considered the various adrenergic antagonists as agents for intravenous regional block. Guanethidine was felt to give the more complete and sustained benefit in treatment, though bretylium was another drug with few side effects in the 1-3 microgram/kilograms doses employed. Because responses were slow to develop and initially less complete, the technique of IV block was thought to have less utility than sympathetic ganglion block as a diagnostic test. Constructive suggestions were offered in seeking to derive search priorities and criteria for clinical diagnosis, grading and treatment responses. These required further definition of the syndrome of RSD and a physiological identification of each of the functional abnormalities which develop. As each of the presentations revealed, our recent advances have led to new concepts which look to have major implications for further study. In response to these demands two subgroups of speakers were assigned to provide written submissions including the consensus of these discussions. They were each felt to be of such importance that separate reports are appended in this volume.

SUMMARY COMMENTS

M. Stanton-Hicks, W. Jänig

FUTURE PERSPECTIVES:
EXPERIMENTAL NEUROBIOLOGICAL RESEARCH
IN REFLEX SYMPATHETIC DYSTROPHY AND
ITS INTERACTION WITH CLINICAL RESEARCH

Wilfrid Jänig and Michael Stanton-Hicks

The question: Can experimental (neurobiological) research contribute to the understanding of reflex sympathetic dystrophy (RSD) and related syndromes in order to improve both diagnosis and therapy?

The answer is without reservation "yes"; however it requires qualification and the hypotheses need testing. The overall animal model for research on pathophysiological mechanisms of RSD does not exist. Research can only be successful if close interaction between bench and clinical investigation is maintained. In fact, most research to date has obtained its impetus from clinical experience. This does not necessarily mean that experimental scientists and clinicians should literally work together, rather it implies they should communicate with each other in common terms. It is imperative, however, that the experimental scientist remains independent as far as experimental design is concerned.

The putative pathobiological processes most likely involved in the genesis of RSD are schematically outlined in Figure 1, and summarized in Table 2, Chapter 6. It is clear that these pathological changes may occur at different levels of integration:

1. The level of the effector organ (vascular and nonvascular elements, neural elements; coupling between afferent and sympathetic axons, interaction between neural, non-neural and environmental influences).

2. The level of the peripheral neurons that connect target tissue with the spinal cord (primary afferent neurons, sympathetic pre- and postganglionic neurons, motorneurons).

3. The level of the spinal cord (in particular the dorsal horn).

4. The supraspinal "centers" that control spinal machinery (brain stem, higher brain areas).

These four levels of integration interact reciprocally by neural and biochemical signals. Changes in the foregoing can perturb the general homeostasis and may in turn lead to those clinical phenomena ascribed to RSD. Many totally unrelated events can induce the same clinical phenomena: trauma with and without nerve lesions, visceral events (e.g., coronary complications), events in the deep somatic domain (e.g., skeletal muscle, tendons, fascia, bone, etc.), and central lesions. It is theoretically possible for clinical phenomena of RSD to be initiated from the neocortex/limbic system without any trauma or lesion. How can one explain the generation of RSD following trivial peripheral trauma? The structure most critical to this answer is the spinal cord, in particular the dorsal horn with its neuronal input systems (cutaneous, deep somatic, visceral; from supraspinal "centers") and its output systems (sympathetic, skeletomotor, to brain stem, to thalamus). When seen in this way, RSD is a neurological disease. The sympathetic outflow is only *one* (though notably an important) component of the syndrome. It is less of a mystery that so many totally unrelated events may bring about the same syndrome. Therefore it is also neither advisable nor rational to focus only on the sympathetic nervous system.

Research Integration

Already mentioned and tacitly accepted during the conference is the premise that basic experimental research on different levels of integration is required if we want to understand the pathophysiology of RSD (pain, abnormalities linked with the sympathetic nervous system, abnormalities linked with the motor system, trophic changes, and psychic abnormalities). Such research is directed on the assumption that the pathophysiology can only be understood if one is willing to understand the normal neurobiology of these systems (psychic processes being indivisible from neurobiology!). Research conducted at a clinical level only, will be unlikely to produce much progress in our understanding of pathophysiological processes. How can one explain those clinical phenomena, that comprise hundreds of publications on patients with RSD, still not yield any consistent concept for diagnosis and therapy?

A: *Basic research should concentrate on the different levels of integration:*

1. Experimental research on animals to study changes of behavior under controlled conditions that have clinical relevance (nerve lesions, chronic inflammation, central lesions; before and after sympathetic blocks; with interventions that alter sympathetic activity; with pharmacological interventions). This leads to "pain behavior models" (1,3,4,6,10; see Chapters 9 and 14 in ref. 5), animal models of trophic changes and animal models of abnormal motor activity.

2. Experimental research on animals to study single neurons (afferent neurons, motorneurons, sympathetic neurons, dorsal horn neurons, etc.) in the context of the whole system. Research on whole systems requires well controlled conditions under anesthesia. The work must focus on mechanisms, at the level of a single neuron, with respect to target organs (blood vessels, sweat glands, skeletal muscle) and in respect to the central control systems. Such research may be directly related to research done on unanesthetized humans using effector organ recordings and microneurography for recording from peripheral neurons (afferent, sympathetic postganglionic, motoraxons) [see Roberts, Chapter 7; Torebjörk, Chapter 9; Blumberg, Chapter 10, see refs. 7-9].

3. Experimental research on isolated systems. This includes *in vitro* work. This should focus on morphological, biochemical and neurophysiological alterations of afferent and efferent neurons after their interaction with target organ changes, on the neuroeffector (predominantly neurovascular) transmission, on the role of afferents in neurovascular transmission to small pre- and postcapillary blood vessels, on the development and mechanisms of coupling between postganglionic and afferent axons in the periphery, and on the interaction between neural, environmental and non-neural elements, etc.

B: *Basic research should be done in close concert with the clinical and psychological research on patients.* This should include:

1. Quantitative work on phenomena, epidemiology, and incidence of RSD.

2. Quantitative work on sensory, motor, autonomic and trophic alterations of RSD using modern methods.

3. Controlled quantitative studies about the efficacy of treatment of RSD (physiotherapy, sympathetic blocks, psychological and behavioral therapy, pharmacological therapy, other supportive therapies) that is time dependent following onset of the symptoms of RSD and related to initiating events (i.e., sensory, autonomic, motor and trophic changes).

4. Studies of psychologic/psychosomatic aspects of RSD. These should focus on the question whether predisposing psychosocial components exist to enhance the development of RSD and second, the psychologic and mental alterations that in turn influence the course of the disease.

Clinical research will create ideas that are only verifiable in basic research and vice versa. Quantitative clinical research by itself should create improved comparative criteria and acceptable standards for diagnosis and treatment of RSD. A practical means of evaluating abnormal function of the sympathetic, motor and sensory systems based on a practical means of evaluating dysfunction should lead to some agreement as to the grading and severity of RSD. Such research should also lead to a common taxonomy.

C: *Basic research on animals that is associated with RSD requires the understanding and support of the medical community.* Experimental research today on integrative systems using anesthetized animals is in grave danger, because of the lack of public support. Only those who are actively involved in clinical research with RSD can provide the type of information for the media, public and government agencies which can assuage community attitudes, in support of basic mechanistic research. The clinician who understands difficulties in the diagnosis and treatment that commonly results in a perpetuation of the patient's pain and suffering, to say nothing of the economic burden, is best placed to assist the basic scientist in his or her dilemma.

If the medical community is unable to reach a consensus in defense of basic research on animals and should there be no financial support of such research there will be little enticement to any young scientist who is willing to do this demanding research.

PROPOSED DEFINITION OF
REFLEX SYMPATHETIC DYSTROPHY

The following definition of Reflex Sympathetic Dystrophy (RSD) represents a synthesis of the many views that were put forward by all who attended the workshop at Schloss Rettershof. The final draft as it appears here is a consensus of these views collated by those below named. It will be submitted in this form to the Subcommittee on Taxonomy of the International Association for the Study of Pain for consideration as being a clinically more precise instrument that that which presently appears in Supplement 3, 1986 of Pain.

Authors:

S. E. Abram, M.D.
H. Blumberg, M.D.
R. A. Boas, M.D.
J. D. Haddox, M.D.
W. Jänig, Ph.D.
H. Kruescher, M.D.

G. B. Racz, M.D.
P. P. Raj, M.D.
W. J. Roberts, Ph.D.
M. Stanton-Hicks, M.D.
M. Zimmerman, M.D.

Definition

A syndrome of continuous diffuse limb pain, often burning in nature, and usually consequent to injury or noxious stimulus, and disuse, presenting with variable sensory, motor, autonomic and trophic changes; causalgia represents a specific presentation of RSD associated with peripheral nerve injury.

Clinical Features

The symptoms and changes spread independently of both the source and site of the precipitating event, presenting with a glove and stocking anatomical distribution. Clinical findings include disturbances of:

> **Autonomic deregulation.** Alterations in blood flow, hyper/hypohydrosis, edema.
> **Sensory abnormalities.** Hypo or hyperesthesia, allodynia to cold and mechanical stimulation.
> **Motor dysfunction.** Weakness, tremor, joint stiffness.
> **Trophic changes.** Skin, hair, nails.
> **Psychologic reactive disturbances.** Anxiety, depression, hopelessness. (As with other chronic pain patients.)

These features manifest diffusely but not necessarily uniformly in the entire distal extremity. They occur at a variable time after the onset of the syndrome, spreading proximally and occasionally to the opposite side as the syndrome progresses. Dominating symptoms are spontaneous pain, swelling, and weakness.

Diagnostic Tests

> **Autonomic.** Bilateral symmetrical multidigital temperature measures by surface thermistors or thermography, show consistent discrepancies (cooler or warmer) on the affected side.
>
> **Sensory.** Lowered thresholds to pinprick, light touch, and cold.
>
> **Motor.** Reduced measures of strength as well as active and passive range of motion.
>
> **Block response.** Sympathetic block usually abolishes diffuse burning pain and allodynia, also raises skin temperature to 35-36°C, and abolishes the vasoconstrictor response to cold stimulation.
>
> **Bone scan.** Three phase scanning shows distinctive, diffuse patterns of increased flow, pooling and delay.

Nonspecific confirmatory tests can be used to further quantify changes and follow progress. These include radiographic densitometry testing of osteopenia, water displacement plethysmography for measures of swelling, plus tests of sudomotor function such as skin conductivity or potentials, or quantitative sweat testing.

Staging

Cases present with qualitative differences in pain intensity and clinical features, which are not necessarily time or stimulus intensity dependent. Patients with this syndrome should be graded according to the intensity of their presenting features, as being mild, moderate or severe in each of the categories of sensory, autonomic and motor changes. Eponymous or causative designations provide no quantitative or therapeutic benefit. Patients with sympathetically maintained pain may show benefit to sympathetic block, but have localized pain distribution with only one or two of the other accompanying hallmarks distinctive of RSD. In time, however, these conditions may evolve into the full syndrome complex.